VOICES
FROM THE
FIELD

First edition, August, 2003.

For more information or to purchase this or other publications, please contact

Human Systems Dynamics Institute
50 East Golden Lake Road
Circle Pines, Minnesota 55014

Phone/Fax: 763.783.7206
Toll free: 866.473.4678
or online at: www.hsdinstitute.org.

ISBN 0-9740498-0-8

WHAT THE EXPERTS SAY...

Kristine Quade, MSOD, JD, Quantum Change Associates, Author of *The Conscious Consultant: Mastering Change from the Inside Out*
> "The next generation of organization development theory and practice will emerge at the intersection of the new sciences and the social sciences. Human systems dynamics is a promising place to start that evolution."

Alan Barstow, Ph.D., Organizational Dynamics, University of Pennsylvania, Union Institute and University Graduate School, Co-Founder of Institute for Interactive Management
> "Human systems dynamics moves beyond organization development to integrate patterns of complexity and nonlinear dynamics. My students and my clients find complexity to be the source of powerful concepts, tools, and techniques."

Michael Quinn Patton, Ph.D., Union Institute and University Graduate School, Author of *Utilization-Focused Evaluation*
> "Eoyang brings together the metaphors of complexity and the practice of organizational change into an action-based praxis that she calls human systems dynamics. It is one of the few applications of complexity to social systems that is more than mere metaphor."

Peter Vaill, DBA, Antioch University, Author of *Learning as a Way of Being: Strategies for Survival in a World of Permanent White Water*
> "Human systems dynamics and the CDE Model for self-organizing systems uncovers the mechanics of the patterns that are familiar to generations of social, political, and organizational professionals. *Voices* presents the principles in accessible ways and provides tools and techniques that anyone can use."

Jack Cohen, Ph.D., D.Sc., University of Warwick, Co-author *The Collapse of Chaos: Discovering Simplicity in a Complex World*

"Ecologists have changed the structure of the subject over the last decade, incorporating complex-systems theory, symmetry-breaking and much new thinking — we nearly understand a few ecosystems now. Glenda Eoyang has dared to do the same for our human organizations; *Voices from the Field* will show you new ways of understanding the ecology of human beings in industrial societies."

Acknowledgements

Emergence only happens when energy is invested in a system. The self-organizing process that generated this book demonstrates the truth of this truism. Many people pooled their energies in this creative process. Thanks to all of them!

In particular I would like to thank Mark Habrel, who birthed the project and gave it a name; Linda Rening, whose sensitive hand brought the authors together without damping their individual voices; Ronda Zimmerschied, who shared her vision and technology to make the ideas manifest.

Special thanks should also go to Royce Holladay, Director of the Network; Dennis Cheesebrow, Director of Services; and the members of the Associates and Science Advisory Boards of the Human Systems Dynamics Institute. With their help, this new organization is facilitating the development of theory and practice in human systems dynamics.

Finally, thanks to our authors. They are explorers of uncharted lands. Their theory and practice, their day-to-day experiences, provide lessons for all of us in creativity and courage.

With sincere thanks for past and hope for future,

Glenda H. Eoyang

Voices from the Field

Table of Contents

Preface: Why this book? Why now?

Glenda H. Eoyang, Ph.D.

The field of human systems dynamics is emerging. Just like the complex phenomena it seeks to understand, this field includes broadly diverse perspectives, multiple levels of organization, complicated histories, and unknowable futures. In spite of its complexity, human systems dynamics offers fruitful new approaches for beginners, as well as experienced theoreticians and practitioners. *Voices from the Field* is intended to contribute to the learning journey of everyone engaged in the work of human systems dynamics.

For those new to the field, *Voices from the Field* provides many possible avenues for further investigation. It defines basic concepts in the contexts of practice and emerging theory. It introduces real people who are learning, using, and teaching the lessons of complexity applied to human systems. It tells the stories of organizations that break free from constraints of outmoded, linear policies and practices.

For those who have studied complexity and social systems, *Voices from the Field* both confirms and challenges basic assumptions. As the field has emerged, each investigator has built a base of assumptions on which to stand. Some of those assumptions will be confirmed, and others will be tested in the stories and perspectives included here.

Theoreticians will see principles of nonlinear dynamics and complexity theory applied in some unorthodox, but useful, ways. By exploring these edges of theoretical foundations, by taking them seriously and exploring their potential, new and innovative options might arise to break through some of the theoretical barriers that have emerged in the field in the past.

Practitioners will find new options for effective action in complex human systems. They may discover new models and tools to integrate into their own practices. At the very least, they will witness how others leverage the patterns of complexity to work more productively with dynamics that occur naturally in social systems of all kinds.

The contributions to *Voices from the Field* were selected to:

- Demonstrate applications of human systems dynamics at individual, group, and institutional levels.

- Represent a wide range of interpretations of complexity and human systems.

- Incorporate emerging theoretical frames, research paradigms, and practices.

- Generate questions and conversation to move the field forward.

Many people contributed to *Voices from the Field,* and the Human Systems Dynamics Institute wishes to thank them all. The authors deserve tremendous thanks for their on-going work with human systems dynamics, their skill in telling their own stories, and their generosity in sharing their work with others. We must also thank all of the writers cited throughout the book. Each, in his or her way, has established the foundations and frameworks within which each of us pursues the work. This book, the Institute, and the field that they support have emerged from the generative relationships among people engaged in shared inquiry. Our thanks go to each of them.

The dynamical interactions among people in the field are generating new models for understanding as well as innovative individual, group, organizational, and community practices. The purpose of *Voices from the Field* is to facilitate and contribute to this process of creative evolution. The book was inspired by the complex dynamics of self-organizing in human systems, which it intends to elucidate. It was designed to demonstrate and apply the best of the working principles that are emerging from the study of dynamic human systems. By following some of the basic principles of complexity, the book reflects the dynamical emergence of the field and of the courageous and curious individuals who pursue the work. This brief introduction articulates some of the principles applied in the creation of the book, but the best way to see the complex patterns as they emerge is to experience them for yourself by reading the wonderfully diverse, energetic, and innovative stories the authors have been generous enough to share.

Whether you begin with stories that match your personal experience and interests, explore the most unfamiliar, or simply read from beginning to end, you will find here rich similarities to, and differences from, your own knowledge and experiences. We hope these differences stimulate new paths of inquiry for you and for the field.

INTRODUCING THE FIELD

HUMAN SYSTEMS DYNAMICS IS THE EMERGING FIELD THAT INTEGRATES COMPLEXITY AND SOCIAL SCIENCES. AS A FIELD OF THEORY AND PRACTICE, IT REFLECTS THE FUNDAMENTAL PATTERNS OF THE COMPLEX AND ADAPTIVE HUMAN SYSTEMS IT STUDIES. GLENDA EOYANG EXPLORES THE UNDERLYING PARADOXES OF SOCIAL SYSTEMS RESEARCH AND PRACTICE AND ARTICULATES HOW HUMAN SYSTEMS DYNAMICS TRANSCENDS THOSE TRADITIONAL DILEMMAS. IN THE PROCESS, SHE BUILDS THE FOUNDATION FOR HUMAN SYSTEMS DYNAMICS AS A VIBRANT AND ENLIGHTENING FIELD OF STUDY AND ACTION.

Human Systems Dynamics: Beyond the Usual Paradoxes

Glenda H. Eoyang, Ph.D.

Beginnings

Beginning in the late 1980s, social scientists and organizational practitioners began to investigate principles of chaos theory and complexity science. The hope was that these new models of nonlinear causality, emergence, and unpredictability would provide a foundation for more realistic models of the dynamics of human systems. Over the last 15 years, as the physical sciences and mathematics uncovered new insights about complex dynamics, social scientists and practitioners developed new ways to think about and work productively in complex human systems (Olson & Eoyang, 2001).

This developmental process has been messy and diffuse. Initially, the openness and ambiguity increased creativity in the field, as each individual discovered unique ways to understand and apply the principles of complexity. As the field developed, however, isolated pockets of theory and practice emerged and threatened to Balkanize the field.

Human systems dynamics is developing as an effort to use the principles of complexity to establish a flexible, resilient, and creative field in which humans at all levels and interests, and systems of all kinds, can benefit from fuller understanding of their underlying dynamics.

Within the framework of human systems dynamics, some of the basic paradoxes of social sciences cease to be differences that make a difference, and new, more generative distinctions emerge as significant. The mission of The Human Systems

Dynamics Institute is to facilitate the development of theory and practice in the field. The Institute's first book, *Voices from the Field,* exemplifies the principles of human systems dynamics in both its process of creation and its content. The following pages describe some of the fundamental underpinnings of human systems dynamics and explain how it is fundamentally different from other approaches to psychological, organizational, and political theory and practice. It includes the following topics:

- The Physical and the Social Sciences
- Exploration and Exploitation
- Theory and Practice
- Part, Whole, and Greater Whole
- Finite and Infinite

The Physical and the Social Sciences

At the simplest and most global level, human systems dynamics is a marriage between the natural sciences of complexity and the social sciences. The complexity sciences have themselves emerged from complicated interdependencies. Mathematics, computer sciences, physics, thermodynamics, chemistry, meteorology, and numerous life sciences have introduced questions about unpredictable and surprising behaviors of natural and information systems. Researchers have identified similar patterns of behavior in radically different contexts, including sensitive dependence on initial conditions, fractal self-similarity, nonlinear interactions, and system-wide patterns that are different from the sum of the parts (Briggs and Peat, 1989; Morowitz, 2002). Each discipline has explored these similar behaviors within its own domain using familiar tools, models, and idioms. Diverse disciplines have also initiated conversations among themselves to explore the similarities that cross traditional practice and research divisions (Cowan, et al., 1994).

Based on the work in the physical sciences, social scientists investigated complex adaptive and emergent behavior at a variety of structural levels (Eoyang, 1997). Individual psychologists, group facilitators, management theorists, political scientists, and others concerned with social behavior have begun to recognize patterns of complex systems in their own domains. They have initiated studies into complexity to develop new theoretical foundations, to explore new practice possibilities, and to test the reliability of their procedures (Dooley, 1996; Goldstein, 1994; Stacey, et al., 2000).

Today these multiple threads of inquiry and application merge into a single field called human systems dynamics. No one knows what this marriage will engender, but scholars and practitioners from various disciplines are engaging with each other to explore options for thought and action when discoveries about complexity are applied to questions about humans and their institutions.

Human systems dynamics practitioners represent many of these diverse threads of inquiry and practice. Theology, community development, psychology, education, management, and many other disciplines are reflected in their work.

Exploration and Exploitation

Human systems dynamics expresses itself in an on-going interaction of exploration and exploitation. Traditionally in the social sciences (especially those with obvious market value such as organization development or management) exploration and exploitation were carefully separated in time and purpose. The old game was simple: "Explore the possibilities; find an innovative approach; and then move into exploitation of the discovery. To exploit a finding to its fullest, package, promote, and protect the discovery." The purpose was to ensure the fullest possible return from the innovation before others gained control over the "intellectual property."

Some genuine innovation resulted, but this approach also generated many pseudo-innovations, slickly packaged and sold to the unsuspecting corporate buyer. As long as an idea or product looked or sounded different enough, it might go under lock and key for the sales push. In the most extreme cases, over-simplification and commercialization of the work diluted its power and interfered with open inquiry and the constructive clash of ideas among explorers in the field.

Based on the principles of nonlinear dynamics and complexity, human systems dynamics assumes that interaction increases value rather than decreases it, so that exploration and exploitation feed on each other throughout the process. The more ideas that are on the table, the more each of us will learn, and the more valuable our work will become. The best way to expand learning is to share it with others. Feeding into their explorations contributes to an ecology of rich inquiry and encourages on-going creation of new ideas and wealth. A system of diverse nonlinear interactions has the potential to generate a whole that is greater than the sum of the parts and for each of the parts to benefit from the richness of the whole.

Voices from the Field demonstrates the benefit of simultaneous exploration and exploitation. Each of the authors made a conscious decision to share "work in progress." Of course they wish to be duly respected and maintain ownership over their own contributions. But this urge is balanced by the desire to share ideas, receive feedback, and contribute to the rich discourse of learning in the field. As the conversation continues, we all—reader and writer—share in the benefits of inquiry that both explores new ideas and exploits old ones.

Theory and Practice

At a more personal and local level, human systems dynamics is an on-going interplay of theory and practice. For generations, people who investigate human systems have faced a difficult dilemma. A model of social systems could be general, or accurate, or simple, but not all three (Weick, 1979). Pure practice usually was specific, accurate, and complicated because it was inextricably connected with the characteristics of a given group, place, and time. Pure theory, on the other hand, was most often general, approximate, and simple because it had to allow for mathematical precision. Thus, theory moved out of the realm of the "real." Most theoreticians and practitioners worked somewhere between these two extremes, making compromises in theoretical rigor to accomplish practical benefits, but each saw the choices as unpleasant compromises.

Human systems dynamics, with its roots in complexity science, makes this dichotomy between theory and practice obsolete. Descriptions of complex systems can simultaneously be specific and general, accurate and approximate, and simple and incredibly complicated.

Principles from complexity can be both specific and general because of the natural self-similarity of complex systems, recognized as fractal structures. Because the patterns of the whole are reflected in each part, it is possible to discover system-wide characteristics by examining local behaviors. Local behaviors may also be discovered in the emergent system-wide patterns. The traditional distinction between general and specific loses relevance as complex systems self-organize into coherent wholes.

Complex systems can be both accurate and approximate, depending on the level of organizational structure under consideration. During the self-organizing process, structures emerge across the system. These emergent patterns are accurate representations of the whole, and they are approximate representations of the parts. At the same time, when the pattern is replicated from whole to part, the system-wide pattern may be an accurate representation of the part as well. Regardless of the degree of resolution, the patterns remain unchanged in these surprising systems and generate descriptive models that are, at the same time, both accurate and approximate.

Finally, complex systems can be simultaneously complicated and simple. Complex systems appear to be complicated, but research and experience indicate that intricate patterns may emerge from a short list of simple rules. Simple rules for relationship and behavior can generate unpredictable and quite complicated behaviors, depending on the environment and initial conditions in which the rules are applied.

These characteristics of complex systems blur the traditional distinctions between practice and theory — specific and general, accurate and approximate, and complicated and simple. So, in the world of human systems dynamics, the line between theory and practice becomes less distinct. The most powerful theory emerges from specific times and places, and the most influential practice draws from simplified models incorporating multiple perspectives and possibilities.

The stories and reflections included in *Voices from the Field* likewise bridge the chasm between theory and practice. Each author has experienced the confluence of the two and created a written representation of the encounter. Some of the stories focus on theory development or testing and relegate practice to merely context or occasion. Others speak primarily of practice, and theory serves as a backdrop in the telling. Each author finds the voice that uniquely reflects his or her experience and, as a reader, you have the opportunity to reflect on your own experiences and consider the ways in which theory and practice intermingle for you.

Part, Whole, and Greater Whole

The emergence of the field of human systems dynamics occurs at a variety of levels. Individuals build cognitive capacity, teams of researchers build new models for theory and practice, the field as a whole establishes new standards of quality. This, too, is true of the complex systems we investigate: Emergence at one level of organization is fed by other levels below or beside it, and feeds into levels above or adjacent to it. For example, rejuvenating cycles within cells revitalize tissues, which contribute to strengthening organs, whole individuals, and, eventually, complete species. At the same time, processes and products at higher organizational levels have obvious influence over lower levels. The same multi-level patterns appear in other complex systems, and the field of human systems dynamics is no exception.

First, the individual is inquiring and learning, experimenting and adapting. Emerging personal theories and practices self-organize as the individual interacts dynamically with the surroundings. Second, the field itself emerges. Defined first in 2001, human systems dynamics is just beginning to settle into a set of shared assumptions, common perspectives, and agreed-upon tools. As individuals share their learning and inquire together, the nature of the field emerges and is reinforced in word and deed. Third, the larger field of complexity and its applications continues to emerge. Individual disciplines dig deeper into their own questions and domains, while the inter-disciplinary conversation continues among traditional disciplines.

Discoveries in human systems dynamics necessarily emerge at all of these levels simultaneously. Developments at one level set the context for developments at other levels. For this to happen efficiently, however, the levels have to be connected. An individual who is isolated from others will not only thwart individual growth, but will also fail to contribute to the development of the whole and the greater whole. If the field of human systems dynamics is not connected directly to individual learning and evolution of the larger field, then it will be threatened with irrelevancy or, even worse, the self-satisfaction that arises from unjustified certainty.

By its very existence, *Voices from the Field* builds connections between and among the many levels of self-organizing patterns in the field of human systems dynamics. Emerging development of individuals, the Human Systems Dynamics Institute, other organizations, and the field as a whole are made interdependent by the creation and the consumption of this book. It builds what Jack Cohen calls "strange loops" among massively entangled self-organizing systems. (Cohen & Stewart, 1994).

The Finite and the Infinite

Human systems like other complex systems are open to their environments, yet they are bounded sufficiently to maintain a shared identity. They are finite at the same time that they incorporate infinite possibilities. Within this paradox lies one of the most powerful engines for evolutionary change. At the same time that the agents in a system are interacting and forming system-wide patterns, new agents enter the system and participate in this and other self-organizing processes. Differences among system agents (old and new) contribute to the richness and resilience of the continually emerging pattern.

The field of human systems dynamics and the individuals and institutions engaged in its evolution must replicate this complicated paradox to remain vital. While holding some ideals and principles in common, we must invite an ever-increasing diversity of perspectives. In the on-going dialogue that is the field of human systems dynamics, difference must be seen as an engine for learning rather than as a threat to survival. While an experience or individual can be seen as complete and whole, it must also be perceived in a fluid connection to others, both local and remote.

This principle, too, shaped the creation of *Voices from the Field*. Each of the articles is complete in itself, yet each is only a segment out of individual or institutional life. The authors are whole and complete reflections of the field, yet many others can and should be likewise engaged. These authors are special because they are here, but they come from a vast community of people who are also building theory and practice in human systems dynamics in response to their own unique challenges.

You, too, can join the journey. Reflect on your theories and practices that emerge out of human systems dynamics, share them with others in a spirit of inquiry and learning. Join the network of learners and teachers who are this emerging field of human systems dynamics and contribute your experiences, insights, and questions to the pattern of human systems dynamics.

Conclusion

Human systems dynamics is an emerging field. *Voices from the Field* introduces the field by sharing multiple views on some of the models and practices that are being generated by individuals around the world.

It also introduces human systems dynamics by using fundamental distinctions of the field in its design and execution. The various disciplines of the writers indicate how multi-disciplinary conversations build a foundation tapestry for the field. The generosity of the authors to share their emerging learnings demonstrates how exploration and exploitation intertwine in a healthy emergent system. The diversity of voices and views articulate the disappearing distinction between theory and practice in human systems dynamics. The integration of diverse individual stories into a single book, and the relationship of that book to the emerging field show how the part, the whole, and the greater whole depend on each other for success. And the paradox of bounding for identity and opening for adaptation establishes one of the primary success criteria for the emerging field. It also serves as an invitation to every reader to explore personal emerging theory and practice and generously share new learnings with others. These human systems dynamics will result in a healthy emerging future for the field of human systems dynamics, and all of us who practice within it.

Glenda H. Eoyang, Ph.D.

Dr. Glenda Eoyang is founding Executive Director of the Human Systems Dynamics Institute, a network of individuals and organizations developing theory and practice in human systems dynamics. She is also President of Chaos Limited, Inc., an organization development and management consulting firm. Dr. Eoyang applies principles of self-organizing systems to help people understand and work productively in unpredictable environments. Since 1988, she has provided training, coaching, and facilitation support to organizations in the public and private sectors. Her areas of specialization include education and training, technology and strategic planning, evaluation, leadership, and whole-system change. She has been an invited lecturer internationally for professional organizations, businesses, and university programs.

She is founder of the Complexity Consortium and a member of the Institute for Coherence and Emergence, the Plexus Institute, and the Teaching/Learning Collaborative. She received her doctorate in Human Systems Dynamics under Donald Klein at The Union Institute and University. Her published works include *Coping with Chaos: Seven Simple Tools, Facilitating Organization Change: Lessons from Complexity Science* (which she wrote with Ed. E. Olson) and numerous articles and lectures.

INDIVIDUAL ADAPTATION

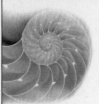

SUPERVISORY RELATIONSHIPS, ESPECIALLY IN TIMES OF ORGANIZATIONAL CHANGE, CAN GENERATE MORE DIFFICULT HUMAN SYSTEMS DYNAMICS THAN ALMOST ANY OTHER CONTEXT. IN THIS THOUGHTFUL STORY, ROYCE HOLLADAY PRESENTS AN INTEGRATION OF THEORY AND PRACTICE THAT CAN UNRAVEL THE CHALLENGES OF INDIVIDUAL ADAPTATION. SHE PULLS TOGETHER CONCEPTS, TOOLS, AND TECHNIQUES FROM THREE SOURCES TO CREATE A UNIQUE AND EFFECTIVE PLAN FOR BUILDING A GENERATIVE RELATIONSHIP WITH HER EMPLOYEE. HER APPROACH IS SUBTLE, POWERFUL, AND APPLICABLE IN A VARIETY OF RELATIONSHIPS.

USING HUMAN SYSTEMS DYNAMICS IN SUPERVISORY RELATIONSHIPS

By Royce Holladay, M. Ed.

A few years ago I worked with a colleague — let's call him George — who had been in his position for a number of years. He was skilled at what he did and was widely respected for his expertise in his field. Additionally George was a warm and friendly individual who was honest and caring in his relationships. It was clear, however, that his full potential remained untapped. He had skills, abilities, and experiences beyond those required for his current position. I was his direct supervisor four of the five years we worked together. In those years, we, along with others on our team, supported each other through a number of organizational challenges. The result was a strong relationship of professional trust and respect.

The organization was experiencing a number of changes, and, as a member of the senior management team, I participated in decisions about reorganizing our services and departments. In some cases we were forced to define new functional roles while eliminating current jobs. Through this process, we identified a position that required the very skills George possessed, and we decided to reassign him.

As his supervisor, I sat down with him to discuss this new assignment. I acknowledged his commitment to the organization and his high standards for his own performance. I explained the new organizational assignment, outlining the rationale behind our decisions and the match between his skills and those we needed in this new position. In the conversation, we discussed supports and resources he would need in the transition. As his friend and colleague, I expressed my understanding that he was not happy about this move and pledged my personal support throughout this transition.

In the following days and weeks, it was obvious that George was angry and hurt by this change of assignments, even as he attacked the challenges of the new role. I kept my promises about training, information, and support, while continuing to reinforce my personal commitment to his success. We met frequently to discuss his challenges and to identify additional supports and resources he needed. After a time, however, he established himself in the role and brought his department to a level of service and performance that far exceeded previous accomplishments. Even more important, he was happy in his job.

About six months after his reassignment, George made an appointment to meet with me. He told me he wanted to thank me for "forcing" this challenge on him. He acknowledged the fit between the job and his skills and expressed his pride in what he had been able to accomplish. He asked me how I had known just what he needed to make this transition and to reach the level of pride and joy he had found in his new position. In response, I reached for a pencil and drew him a picture.

Self-organization as Frame

In the field of human systems dynamics, different theorists have studied self-organization. Various perspectives describe the process, examine the conditions, and define the constraints that determine what happens in self-organization. Ralph Stacey, Jeffrey Goldstein, and Glenda Eoyang are three theorists whose descriptions are highly complementary, deceptively simple, and clearly scalable in an organization.

Ralph Stacey describes what happens in a system as its environment becomes less certain and as its agents move further from agreement (Stacey, 1996). He uses a matrix to describe the dimensions the system experiences and their relative impacts on the process. Zimmerman, Lindberg, and Plsek applied his matrix to decision making (Zimmerman, Lindberg, and Plsek, 2001).

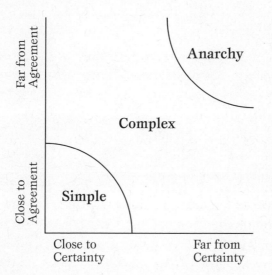

In this diagram, the x-axis reflects a continuum of **certainty,** the degree to which cause and effect linkages can be determined. When issues or decisions are close to certainty, cause and effect linkages are clear. Relationships, dependencies, and issues can be described as straightforward and simple. When issues are less certain, it is more and more difficult to identify direct causes. When issues are far from certainty, there is no way to identify a specific cause in any given issue.

The y-axis represents **agreement**—the degree to which the participants in the decision or issue agree on what is happening and what needs to happen. In situations with high agreement, participants all see the issues in the same way and agree about actions to take as well as the likely outcomes of those actions. As agreement decreases, participants in the decision making are further apart in their opinions, and decisions become more complex. At the point where there is little or no agreement between the participants, behavior of the group becomes random and unpredictable.

As the matrix shows, when issues are close to certainty and close to agreement, the decision is simple. For example, in established procedures, employees can be certain of actions to take, and they agree on those actions. When employees are far from certainty and far from agreement, anarchy reigns. Not only do they not know what to do, they cannot find agreement about how to define their situation.

The area in the center is where issues are defined as complex—the zone of complexity. Zimmerman, et. al., point out that in this area, creativity and innovation are at their peak (Zimmerman, et. al., 2001). This zone of complexity is the area where self-organization occurs—patterns emerge as the system moves toward predictability and agreement.

I knew that George would be operating in this zone as he moved into his new position. Some levels of agreement and certainty existed— the job was known, there were rules and regulations he needed to fulfill, and resources were available. However he had no systems in place, he was not sure of the system-wide impacts of this area, and he did not know all that was required of him. There was enough uncertainty and enough lack of agreement to put George into that zone of complexity. I knew that he would have to operate there for a while, and that he would need tools and various kinds of support to function there successfully.

With George operating in this zone of complexity, I knew that he would be in the process of "self-organizing" in this new position. I needed to find a way to support his work and assure that he was able to self-organize in ways that assured his success and productivity.

Self-organization as Process

In his work, Jeffrey Goldstein describes his theory about how systems organize (Goldstein, 1994). His work is with organizations as they move far from equilibrium, helping them to re-establish their systems and patterns of operating. He essentially provides a description of what happens in a system during the process of self-organization, and that description is clearly scalable from the organizational level to the individual who is experiencing change.

When systems are operating at or near equilibrium, boundaries are established and understood, the agents within the system know what they are to do, and outcomes are generally predictable. For the individual, life is relatively easy, not much is changing, and there are few surprises.

At some point, a system experiences an "event" that throws it into a state far from equilibrium. In this state, the old boundaries are gone, the agents don't know what to do, and there is little that is predictable in the system. When these boundaries explode completely, the system experiences the "anarchy" described by Stacey. There is little that is certain, and agreement is absent. For individuals, this kind of system can result from a powerful change in their lives — death of a family member, significant change in their work situation, or a life-threatening illness or event. When put into such a situation, individuals feel a total loss of control and a lack of connection to their past or to others in their world. The dominant feelings are anger and fear, and their first reactions are to seek ways to regain some semblance of control and/or connection.

In such a system state, eventually, the agents begin to organize themselves around particular issues or expectations, and patterns of behavior begin to emerge. As these patterns become discernable, more agents are attracted to them, and the system begins to organize itself. On the Stacey diagram, these organizations are moving into the zone of complexity. There is a degree of certainty and the agents can find some common areas of agreement. Goldstein refers to this development of new patterns of behavior as self-organization. Individuals begin their own self-organizing processes as they find ways to regain the level of control they seek.

This description of self-organization applies at both the system (group) level as well as at the level of the individual within the group. Individuals who are in situations that are far from agreement and far from predictability experience the same disequilibrium that Stacey and Goldstein describe for the entire system. The self-organizing principle is scaled to the individuals' levels, with patterns emerging from their own personal experiences and from the support they find from others in their environments.

It is at this point of self-organization that the system—or the individual within the system—is most vulnerable. If the patterns that are identified and amplified are healthy and adaptable, the system is able to continue to build toward its original purpose and it is sustainable. On the other hand, if the patterns are destructive and maladaptive, the system will not thrive. Individuals at this stage may find ways to survive and move forward, or they may succumb to fear and anger, which then generate destructive patterns in their lives.

George was operating in the zone of complexity, and I realized he would be experiencing significant self-organization as he adjusted to the new position and established structures and operational procedures in his new role. He needed to re-order his world and establish his own patterns and systems. His initial reaction was so volatile that he could easily have embraced the anger and fear as a way of existing in his new position.

Like most committed employees, he so strongly identified with his work that the reassignment left him with questions about his own efficacy, about his experiences in the system, and about his perceptions of the professional relationship we had developed. He was embarrassed among his colleagues because he perceived — and imagined that they would perceive — that this reassignment was because his past performance had not been adequate. Because the tasks we assigned him had not been well organized or accepted within the system previously, he believed that this was our attempt to get him to leave the organization. None of these perceptions could have been further from the truth. In his anger and fear, however, George — like any other human in such a situation — decided that they were true.

I knew he was "self-organizing" and that I needed to support him in finding healthy, adaptive ways of dealing with this change. Because I saw his self-organization as a process, my challenge was to identify the types of tools and resources he needed to be able to navigate this transition and establish the systems he needed.

Self-organization as Map

Glenda Eoyang has developed a model describing the conditions that influence the speed, path, and direction of self-organization. The Eoyang CDE Model is a powerful tool that shows leaders how they can influence the placement, shape, and power of the patterns that emerge as their systems change in the process of self-organization. The three conditions that must be considered are the **container,** the **significant differences,** and the **exchanges.**

The **container** sets the bounds for the self-organizing system. It defines the "self" that is organizing. The container may be physical, like a geographic location; organizational, for instance a department; or conceptual; as in the case of the purpose or identity. It is within this container that new relationships and structures emerge from the interactions that occur.

There may be different containers at work at any given time. Changes in an organization may affect parts of the organization that are in different locations or even different areas within the same building. There may be containers that are departmental or hierarchical within the organization. Conceptual containers are the most difficult to discern. The organization's mission is the most obvious conceptual container, but Eoyang points out that professional, personal, psychological, and cultural containers also shape the behaviors of people in every environment.

The **significant differences** cause primary patterns to emerge during the process of self-organization. These patterns arise as the differences are reflected and reinforced by the other agents in the system. When the reinforcement is positive, those differences are amplified and increased or multiplied in a system.

As an example, when everyone pays attention to and shares the negative gossip in a group, its power grows until it permeates the culture. On the other hand, negative reinforcement takes away the power or diminishes the difference until it disappears. If the members of a group ignore negative rumors, they are soon forgotten and lose their power to do damage.

Transforming exchanges form the connections between agents in the system. These exchanges can take the form of money, time, information or any other resources that fuel the system. Whatever the resource may be, as it flows from agent to agent, each is transformed in some way, creating patterns of change that lead to the adaptability of the system.

Feedback is an example of a transforming exchange. One individual observes the performance of another and learns more about the work that is done. That person then shares feedback about the performance, changing the perception and awareness of the person who was observed.

These cannot be considered in a reductionistic view. The conditions and all that they convey are massively entangled. It is crucial to remember that any shift in one of these conditions can bring about change in the others. By influencing or changing one of the conditions of self-organization, the process itself can be altered to produce a different result. Leaders who understand this are able to identify critical points in their organizations where small adjustments, through the process of self-organization, cause change throughout the system. Similarly, leaders who understand this can recognize that even a small unexpected change in one area of their organization has the potential to cause dramatic shifts in all areas.

As organizations and individuals experience change, they are self-organizing in response to the alterations they perceive in their environments. When difficulties and organizational challenges arise, leaders can identify which condition is most affected. For instance, as organizations grow quickly, newer employees often can feel disconnected, without a real commitment to the direction or mission of the organization. When leaders perceive this "container" issue, they can take steps to amplify the connectedness to direction of the organization. Just a small change in this area, can reduce the differences between the "old" and "new" employees, and strengthen the communications (exchanges) between them. Similarly, by emphasizing the similarities of the employees or by making slight changes in the exchanges that happen, those "new" employees can be brought in and made to feel a part of the system.

When leaders understand these conditions and their interdependencies, they know that small steps in important areas can yield significant progress.

To support George in his transition into this new position and into his new role, I knew that I would need to influence his personal process of self-organization. However I knew that I would not be able to do this alone. I needed his input and participation in "mapping" out the process he would follow in his own self-organization. I knew that map needed to influence his personal process of self-organization without interfering in his growth into the position, and the Eoyang CDE Model showed me where I needed to focus my attention. In preparing to engage him in the process of planning for his transition, I identified the container, the differences, and the exchanges that could influence his self-organization toward the productive, committed employee I knew him to be.

Self-organization as Tool

The Eoyang CDE Model describes those conditions that influence self-organization, and it is easily applied at the organizational level. Scaling those conditions, however, to the level of the individual calls for a mid-level abstraction that refines the focus and provides a more specific guide for individual self-organization. Looking in the frame of Goldstein's perspective, this requires consideration of those factors that draw individuals together to initiate patterns in their work.

It is the leader's responsibility to assure that these factors are addressed in ways that assure the emergence of productive patterns. By understanding the factors, the leader can identify supports and exchanges that will amplify desired interactions and behaviors. Supportive relationships, honest feedback, training and development, straightforward information, and a clearly stated organizational purpose are very simple examples of ways to amplify what is desired.

Conversely, the leader may also reduce interactions and behaviors that may limit or prevent productivity. Ignoring negative behavior and limiting the spread of misinformation are just two examples of ways that leaders can dampen undesired activities.

Individuals are complex beings, bringing with them their experiences, skills, and perspectives as they enter into an organization. What are the discernable factors in the work environment that define productive patterns within the context of the organization? Those factors are **relationship, efficacy,** and **accountability** and are reflected in each of the conditions identified in the Eoyang CDE Model.

Humans are social beings, and to be healthy they need to relate to others and to feel safe in those **relationships.** This means they need to relate to the organization, to the work they have to do, and to the people with whom they work. Productive patterns emerge when the individual's values and goals are aligned with those of the organization; when the work that is to be done has meaning; and when people who work together are able to communicate effectively and efficiently.

It only makes sense that people who are confident of their skills and have mastered their work are happier in their jobs and are better able to contribute to the goals of the organization. Professional development, on-going feedback, individual recognition, and remuneration are some ways that organizations reinforce **efficacy** among their employees to amplify the patterns of performance that are necessary for success.

Accountability is the ability to be responsible and answerable for outcomes. Often in today's culture, the word accountability is used to indicate blame or cause. In this sense, however, it refers to an individual's inherent need and ability to "step up" and take responsibility for contributing to the organization. The first requirement of accountability is clearly articulated expectations and job descriptions. People can and will be accountable for their work when they clearly understand the scope of their responsibilities, the standards against which their work will be measured, and their relative position or responsibility in the organization.

Each of the conditions listed in the Eoyang model gives rise to patterns that are affected by all three factors. For individuals, container issues—the boundaries in the system—are affected by all three factors, with efficacy within the system being the strongest. It is the individual's efficacy within the system that establishes the strongest boundaries, while relationships in the system and accountability also influence container issues. When considering the significant differences at this level, the individual's accountability is fore-grounded, with efficacy and relationships also influencing those issues. Finally, within transforming exchanges, relationships are brought out first. The following table reflects these interdependencies.

Conditions that Influence Self-organization	Factors that define productive patterns within a system (with major factor in bold)
Container	**Efficacy,** Accountability, Relationships
Significant Differences	Efficacy, **Accountability,** Relationships
Transforming Exchanges	Efficacy, Accountability, **Relationships**

As leaders examine and look for ways to influence the conditions of self-organization at the individual level, they need to consider the factors of relationship, efficacy, and accountability in each and answer the following question, "How can I support this individual to move toward increased agreement and certainty in the current situation?"

As George and I planned for his transition, we looked for ways to address each of these factors. I engaged him and others in conversations that addressed the factors and looked for ways to meet the needs he identified. From those conversations, he and I mapped out a plan of action for his transition.

Container Issues

- *I knew that his relationship to the organization was strong. He was committed to the mission and purpose, and had spent his life in this line of work and knew that he could do it. (Factor—Efficacy)*

- *George honestly believed in the value of the position that we had created, even though he did not want to take it on. I knew that I had to continue to take steps to reinforce his commitment and belief in the position. (Factor — Accountability)*

- *Our own personal professional relationship was strong. Our mutual trust and respect contributed to his ability to move forward in spite of his anger and fear. (Factor — Relationship)*

Significant Differences Issues

- *I worked with him to write a full job description and performance standards so that we were both clear on his accountabilities and measures of excellence. (Factor — Accountability)*

- *George was strongly related with others in the organization, and it was critical that he not be perceived to lose status as a result of this change. Consequently I made sure that every communication about this shift, whether written or spoken, addressed his value to the organization, the need for his skills in this new and critical area, and his ability to make this change. (Factor — Relationship)*

- *In spite of his many skills, there were gaps in George's knowledge about this specific role. We sought out training opportunities and information to be sure he was able to accomplish the job, and we invited experts in to coach him and assist him in designing his operational systems. (Factor — Efficacy)*

Transforming Exchanges Issues

- *I continued to express my personal professional support and to offer my friendship, in the face of his anger and frustration. (Factor—Relationship)*

- *We met on a weekly basis and my door remained open to him for support in problem solving and resource allocation. (Factor—Efficacy)*

- *We used his performance standards and the operational outcomes and designed a feedback and evaluation system that would help him assess his own progress as well as his overall contributions to the organization. (Factor—Accountability)*

As we moved through that first six months, I watched him blossom and grow into the role and make it his own. The process was not free of setbacks and frustrations, but at each challenge, we worked through his plan and continued to move forward. Then when he came in that evening and asked me how I had known that he would be successful in this position, I reached for my pencil and drew the following diagram for him.

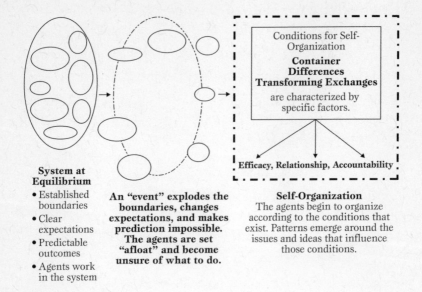

System at Equilibrium
- Established boundaries
- Clear expectations
- Predictable outcomes
- Agents work in the system

An "event" explodes the boundaries, changes expectations, and makes prediction impossible. The agents are set "afloat" and become unsure of what to do.

Self-Organization
The agents begin to organize according to the conditions that exist. Patterns emerge around the issues and ideas that influence those conditions.

George came to see that when we reassigned him, the boundaries of his professional life exploded and left him at loose ends, not knowing what to expect, what he could rely on, or who he was in the organization. By the time I had drawn the final phase of the diagram, he was able to list the steps we had taken to address the various factors and conditions.

Supporting Self-organization—One-on-One

When self-organization occurs at the individual level, there are too many issues to address, too many possibilities to consider, and too many choices to make without some sort of tool that helps to examine the situation as it is occurring. Too often time and energy are spent on random and unconnected actions that do little to move the individual forward. This visual representation, based on the work of Stacey, Goldstein, and Eoyang, along with my own experiences, provides a guide to address individuals' needs as they proceed through transitions.

Planning tools can be developed to help focus discussions and to identify steps that provide meaningful support to individuals.

In today's quickly changing business landscapes, this is the task of supervision: to support individuals as they self-organize in response to changes in their work environments. Change in today's organizations is a fact of life, and human systems dynamics provides a conceptually sound approach to building understanding and skills to meet the challenges that confront workers on a daily basis.

Royce Holladay, M.Ed.

Royce Holladay launched her teaching career in 1979, and has worked as a school district administrator since 1989 in Texas, North Carolina, and Washington. In those years, she used the concepts of complexity in her work on school reform, as well as in working to improve operational systems within school districts. With extensive experience in Special Education, she has worked with staff members at the district and state levels to develop effective programs and systems to meet the needs of diverse learners.

Her current work revolves around making the principles and concepts of human systems dynamics accessible and useful to those who want their organizations to perform to high standards of effectiveness and efficiency. She works with the Human Systems Dynamics Institute as Director of the Network and as Interim Director of The Foundation. In those capacities, she publishes PATTERNS, the monthly newsletter of the Human Systems Dynamics Institute. She provides customer service and support to the Associates and visitors to the HSD Institute website.

Royce also works with the Teaching/Learning Collaborative, a non-profit organization whose mission is to facilitate collaborative research about teaching/learning as transformation. Launching in September of 2003, this action-oriented think tank will use social networks for collaborative research and action around transformational teaching and learning.

As a free-lance writer and consultant, Royce works with a variety of individuals and groups. In her spare time, she pursues her other passions as artist, novelist, and poet.

J. GWEN KENNEDY IS A CONSULTANT'S CONSUL-
TANT. IN HER PRACTICE, AS IN THIS CHAPTER, SHE
INTEGRATES A PROFOUND UNDERSTANDING OF
THEORY, A PRACTICAL CONNECTION TO HER CLIENTS, AND A
REFLECTIVE VIEW OF HERSELF AND HER PRACTICE. AS A
CONSCIOUS PRACTITIONER OF COMPLEXITY IN HUMAN SYSTEMS,
GWEN SHARES THREE CONCRETE WAYS IN WHICH COMPLEXITY
HAS TRANSFORMED HER PERSPECTIVE AND HER BUSINESS.
WHETHER YOU PRACTICE OD OR SOME OTHER FIELD, WHETHER
YOU ARE INDEPENDENT OR ASSOCIATED WITH A CONGLOMERATE,
HER INSIGHTS WILL HELP YOU THINK ABOUT WHAT IT MIGHT
MEAN TO INTEGRATE HUMAN SYSTEMS DYNAMICS INTO YOUR
DAILY LIFE OF WORK AND LEARNING.

APPLICATIONS FOR THE SOLE PRACTITIONER

By J. Gwen Kennedy, Ph.D.

I sit in my office pondering an e-mail I have just received. A colleague is asking if I want to contribute a chapter to her next book, *Voices from the Field*. I have two questions: What can I contribute? and Should I spend time writing when I need to be pursuing billable hours? You see, I am in one of those stages that my financial planner so accurately describes as "paranoia periods." I have been a successful, independent, organization-and-staff development consultant in Alaska since 1986. Yet I still worry when work slows down and the future feels uncertain. At this moment, I am even more worried than usual because I have decided to buy a piece of property bordering my parent's home back in Virginia. I will need to tap into my savings to make the down payment. I ponder what I should do. Then I realize that perhaps by writing about how complexity science has influenced my life, I might find the confidence and comfort this new perspective has given me. And so I begin.

Book after book and article after article in the area of complexity science speaks to a new style of leadership, to the emergence of innovative organizations, and of efforts to create large, complex adaptive systems. As a Ph.D. and scholarly practitioner, I wanted to test the theory and concepts before I offered them as part of my consulting practice. Yet, as a sole practitioner and small business person, I didn't have access to the traditional organizational relationships or structure to test new leadership principles and organizational development strategies. I decided to draw from the concepts of complexity.

If indeed complex systems are scalable, then the theory should be applicable regardless of the size of the system.

With this in mind, I set out to test the theory, principles, and concepts of complexity science on my own, complex system—myself. As a result, I found a language to describe what I had been experiencing and understanding at an intuitive level. I found a world view that helped me to reduce the stress and anxiety that often comes with the pressure to predict and control outcomes. I found a way of viewing my own life as I would view the rhythms and patterns of nature. And I found a way to understand chaos and uncertainty that gave me confidence that we can and will find a way.

Resonating with the Theory

Complexity science, with its focus on emergence, self-organization, inter-dependencies, unpredictability and nonlinearity, provides a world view that goes beyond the Newtonian science perspective of linear, cause-and-effect relationships, mechanistic efficiency and reliability, dissection and reduction, predictability, and control. The difference in focus helped me to understand the tension I felt when others tried to manage all of life as if it were a project. Complexity science gave me a way of looking at the whole without being overwhelmed by the massively entangled issues. Instead of trying to understand the situation from a snapshot in time, I began to view my own business and my client systems as multi-dimensional movies—as life itself. Complexity science helped me to make sense of the non-linearity and the unpredictability of my consulting practice.

The term complex adaptive systems implies several distinct qualities within a system:

1. A great number of connections between a wide variety of elements

2. The capacity to alter or change, i.e., the ability to learn from experience

3. A set of connected or interdependent things — independent agents

(Zimmerman, 2001, p. 8). Well, these descriptors surely resonated with my life. The boundaries around my "system" were not as clearly identifiable as an office building or an organization chart, but the elements were all there.

After living and working for over 22 years in Anchorage and having completed a doctoral program with students and faculty from around the world, I have a fairly extensive network. My clients range from Alaska Native village corporations to Fortune 500 global organizations and include government and non-profit entities. I have also experienced a variety of challenges in the last 22 years of my professional career including three business closures, multiple business ventures, a boom-bust economy, and re-inventing my career at least seven times. I am now working on my eighth transformation. My practice easily meets the criteria for a complex adaptive system.

Locating myself within the descriptors and definitions, I felt even more and more connected to the theory. I then sought practical ways to apply the theory to my consulting practice and my everyday life. Three areas, in particular, resonated for me:

1. Strategic Planning

2. Decision Making

3. Simple Rules

Applications in Strategic Planning

Since starting my practice in 1986, I have developed and implemented annual business plans. Each year I have adapted to the changes in Alaska's natural resource-based economy, changes in my client base, and changes in my clients' requests. In contrast to larger markets, my client base and options for growth are limited by:

- The number of employers in Anchorage with over 200 employees

- The understanding of and the valuing of organization development among potential clients

- The expectation that expertise could only be found out of state

- When I tried to expand my practice outside of Alaska, I found just the opposite challenge: Why hire an OD consultant from Alaska?

To meet these challenges, it became essential that I develop a great number of connections across a variety of industries, government agencies, and non-profit organizations. I had to adapt to different organizational cultures and business environments. To provide my clients with the best information and resources, and to expand my practice outside of Alaska, I had to connect with other consultants inside and outside of Alaska. Many of these consultants were like me, independent or small business people.

Each year my business did well and often better than the year before, despite numerous downturns in the economy and a changing business landscape. Each year in review, I smiled at the flip charts and notes from my annual strategic planning process. Some of it had happened, but much of what had happened was unexpected and unplanned.

When I started my own consulting practice, I had done a business plan and a SWOT analysis—the identification of strengths, weaknesses, opportunities, and threats. Over the years I progressed to the appreciative inquiry approach, which included a review of past successes. I always included a visioning process and developed a task list and timeline with objectives to achieve goal(s). Over time I added an analysis of existing and needed resources and the identification of people I needed for my support system. I created mind maps and charts. I created to-do lists and prioritized the tasks. I figured that if I had clear goals and objectives, stayed focused, and worked hard, I could achieve all that I set out to do.

As I better understood complexity science, I began to look at the history of my business practice through a different set of lenses. I could link my visioning and my strategic plan to some of my successes. But the reality was that I got contracts and work requests because I was in the right place at the right time and knew the right people. Much of it was unplanned and unexpected. Things often happened almost magically with everything seeming to fall into place. I could work hard and I did, but my solitary actions were not making things happen; my relationships with others were making things happen. While the mind map and visioning posters still hung on my wall, the strategic planning charts and to-do lists soon got lost in the emerging plies of paperwork. I would not look at them again until the end of the year, and then I would smile, knowing something else was going on besides making and adhering to a plan.

I began to think of the stories that I told others about how I became an entrepreneur and later started my consulting practice and how it continues to grow. One of my favorites is about how I have tried to leave Alaska on two separate occasions. I had committed to leaving, put my home up for sale, bought a new vehicle more suited for the Lower 48, and did the research on where I wanted to relocate. Both times, a client called and asked if I would help on a new and unique program for their organization. Both times, I explained that while confident I could do the work, I wasn't an expert in the area. Each time the client had insisted that they too were confident that I could do the job and that I was the person they wanted. Alaska had become my community and my learning grounds. My relationships were the key to my business success, not some strategic plan.

So I began to rethink strategic planning from a complexity science perspective.

- I looked for patterns and trends within my own practice and within the consulting field and the economy.

- I focused on relationships, making an effort to further develop existing relationships, to build new relationships, and to reflect on the potential role I could play in connecting resources and serving as an expert in a particular area.

- Instead of working first on a plan, I looked at what resources and connections I had and what I could facilitate.

- I began to include others in my learning experience as I dived into complexity science.

- I relied more on mapping my environment and revisiting that map to see how things had changed. The mind-mapping exercise became more of a storyboard process — a moving picture rather than a snapshot.

- I looked for the underlying success factors for my business, the key relationships, and the emerging requests.

- I tested assumptions and engaged clients more in dialogue than marketing activities.

Most of this shift has actually been an acknowledgment and re-alignment of who I am rather than a change in how I run my business. I have let go of adding efforts to try to control and predict my business outcomes. I have given greater voice to my intuition and observations. I have become more interested in watching what is emerging on the changing landscape — within my community, my clients, and my own life.

So now, at the beginning of each year, instead of doing a SWOT analysis or setting clear goals and objectives with tasks, resources, and timelines, I ask questions. These are the questions I am currently asking myself:

- What does the landscape look like and where do I currently fit and want to fit in that landscape?

- What patterns of needs am I seeing within my client requests and discussions?

- What are my key relationships: who are my connectors, salespeople, and expert resources?

- How does this link with my core values and personal drivers?

- What additional question would be meaningful?

I still do a to-do list and comparative charts. I value facts and data. They are useful tools. But I am looking at my business practice through a different set of lenses and thus looking at the facts and data differently. I am looking not so much for the answer but for the good question to ask. I am also experiencing my world with less stress and more excitement.

Applications for Decision Making

Understanding complexity science gives me a better understanding of chaotic, complex, and unpredictable situations. Yet all of my life is not chaotic. I still have to pay bills on a scheduled basis. I need regular income in order to pay those bills. And much of my life really does seem to operate in a linear, controllable, and independent way. I am aware of the premise that within order there is chaos and within chaos there is order. I know that there were differences in degree of order and chaos. However, it was Glenda Eoyang's and Ed Olson's Decision-Making Model that provided me a useful tool for managing day-to-day decisions. In the spirit of emergence, I have added some tables to their model, which had been inspired by Ralph Stacey's Agreement and Certainty Matrix, to meet my own needs. I have also used this model to help managers see the lessons to be learned from complexity science.

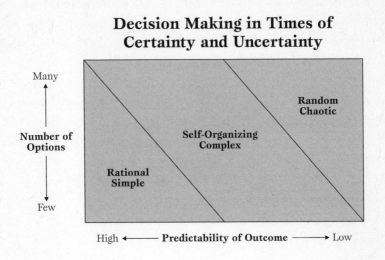

Decision Making in Times of Certainty and Uncertainty

Many ↑

Number of Options

Few ↓

Random Chaotic

Self-Organizing Complex

Rational Simple

High ←——— **Predictability of Outcome** ———→ Low

The model is built upon two axes, one the degree of predictability and the other the number of options. A situation may move along these axes. Some situations may have multiple components—rational, self-organizing, and random.

The rational decision-making process shown below is the most representative of Western minds and habits. It is the foundation of much of management and leadership training. Rational thought is the underlying assumption for tools of project management, root cause analysis, progressive disciplinary action, performance evaluation programs, and traditional strategic planning processes. This perspective is important and helps us function in most aspects of our lives.

Rational Decision-making Process

Language we use	• Who is in charge? • What are your selection criteria? • It's a simple yes or no — one of two or three options. • All I need is to set clear priorities.
Focus	• Goals, tasks, and timelines
Questions to Ask	• What am I trying to achieve? Desired outcomes? Added value? • What needs to be done first, next, last? • How much time and resources will it take? • What should I do?
Tools	• Project Management: goals, objectives, timelines, tasks, accountabilities • Priority Matrix • To-do Lists • Multi-tasking and concurrent engineering • Delegating
How we evaluate	• Ability to accomplish desired outcomes. • Estimated and actual dollars spent, time saved. • Lessons learned from previous experiences, projects.

In contrast, the self-organizing decision-making process (shown on the table below) is the approach grounded in the principles of complexity. The role of leadership then is to work within or change the boundaries of the system or the container, to better understand and benefit from the significant differences, and to facilitate transforming exchanges. This perspective focuses on the movement of the system and its emerging patterns rather than on a specific event.

Self-organizing Decision-making Process

Language we use	• Everything is falling into place/falling apart. • Others are taking the ball and running with it. • There is electricity in the air, excitement. • Trust in the process.
Focus	• Relationships
Questions to Ask	• What difference makes a difference? • What small thing can I do that could have a huge impact? • Where are the energy and resources? • How can I serve as a connector to make things happen?
Tools	• Identifying and working the container, significant differences, and transforming exchanges. (See Olson and Eoyang) • Skillful discussions and dialogue. • Teaming on projects. Leveraging relationships and resources. • Establishing simple rules.
How we evaluate	• Flow of energy, information, and resources. • Adaptability of the system. • Emergence of desired or undesired behaviors.

Finally, the random decision-making process (see the table below) applies to those times of increasing uncertainty and low predictability of outcomes. This process is helpful when we absolutely don't know what to do. When we understand how random, chaotic events are a part of the complexity of life, we can suspend judgment until we begin to see patterns.

Random Decision-making Process

Language we use	• It is difficult to fully comprehend what is happening. • There are no rules…this is uncharted territory. • No one seems to be in charge. • I have no idea what I should do. I am just taking one day at a time.
Focus	• Emerging patterns and strange attractors
Questions to Ask	• What patterns am I observing? • Where is there agreement or common ground? • What happens if I try this? • What else can I try?
Tools	• Mapping emerging patterns of behaviors. • Expanding or contracting the view. • Dialogue and reflective observations. • Trying something; observing and responding to the reaction.
How we evaluate	• Ability to move into self-organizing activities. • Gut level reaction. • Reaction of others.

This decision-making model helps me to assess my situation and decide what action to take. It also helps me to set realistic expectations, focus only on value-added activities, and ultimately reduces stress in my life.

Applications of Simple Rules

One of the premises of complexity science is that simple rules shape the behavior of complex systems. So what simple rules have guided my complex system? I looked back over my life to see what guided my decisions during times of increasing uncertainty and complexity. I remembered times in my life when I made a difficult decision and it changed the direction of my life, dramatically. Some examples include:

- Deciding to travel through India and Nepal alone when my travel partner dropped out

- Deciding to start our own company when the IRS came into the office at 4:00 pm and announced that it was taking over, and we were all immediately out of a job

- Deciding to start a doctoral program when I was unemployed and had no cash reserves

- Deciding to start my own consulting practice when my employer of three months decided to relocate to Seattle

- Deciding to take a four month leave of my consulting practice and go to Latvia during the breakup of the Soviet Union to pursue business and educational joint ventures.

There were many other crossroads that I came to, most when I had limited financial resources, was on my own, and felt a high degree of risk and uncertainty.

As I thought about simple rules, I was interested in what gave me the courage to act. What core values helped me choose my direction? From these reflections I identified my simple rules:

1) Always go for the learning experience.

2) Have faith—there will always be enough money.

3) Respect and value others.

4) Be innovative and practical.

These simple rules are my values in action-verb form. These simple rules guide my actions, help me set priorities, and give me confidence that I am on my personal path.

The review of how complexity science has impacted my life has given me new energy and new focus. The simple rules, the decision-making process model, and the different approach to strategic planning, have helped me focus my energy and resources to support the emergence of my own, self-organizing, complex adaptive system. The decision to share my story has revitalized my journey. Once again, the lens of complexity science has given me insight into my world and helped me to be more confidence and effective.

J. Gwen Kennedy, Ph.D.

J. Gwen Kennedy, Ph.D. has been a consultant in human and organizational systems since 1986. She is experienced in designing organization change activities, facilitating group processes, customizing training programs, and coaching individuals. As a scholarly practitioner, she is passionate about translating new theoretical concepts into everyday use and finding simple interventions that make for meaningful differences in complex systems.

She has consulted to a full spectrum of organizations ranging from village to global corporations, and government and non-profit organizations. Her work has taken her from remote areas of Alaska to the international business community of Geneva, Switzerland.

Her work has included:

- Complex systems analysis and organizational change
- Coaching managers and professionals in problem analysis, strategic decision making, and relationship building
- Training and human resource development programs
- Career management

She has worked with all levels of organizations and in a variety of professional fields including engineering, IT, social services, and healthcare.

Gwen holds a Ph.D. in Human and Organizational Systems and an M.A. in Human Development from the Fielding Institute in Santa Barbara, California. She has a B.S. in Political Science from St. Andrews Presbyterian College in Laurinburg, North Carolina.

TEAM ADAPTATION

WHY DO SOME GROUPS WORK TOGETHER WELL WHILE OTHERS STRUGGLE WITH INTERNAL AND EXTERNAL DISSENT? WHAT BUILDS COHESION IN A WORKING GROUP? HOW CAN FACILITATORS AND MEMBERS OF GROUPS ENCOURAGE INTERACTIONS THAT LEAD TO COORDINATED ACTION? GAYLE BYOCK RESPONDS TO THESE QUESTIONS AND A HOST OF OTHERS IN FRESH AND THOUGHTFUL WAYS. HER GIFT OF METAPHOR AND HER EXPERIENCE WITH HUMAN SYSTEMS LEAD HER TO REFLECT ON THE NATURE OF GROUP COHERENCE. IN THIS PIECE, SHE SHARES A FUN AND FUNCTIONAL TECHNIQUE TO HELP A GROUP ESTABLISH A FOUNDATION OF SHARED MEANING.

CATCH PHRASES TO SPEED THE PROCESS FROM A GROUP'S EMERGENCE TO ITS SELF-ORGANIZATION

By Gayle Byock

"The power of the complexity approach is that it provides language, metaphors, and approaches that embody your best intuitions about how individuals and organizations operate. When these intuitions are articulated, they can be optimized, shared, and used to their best advantage." (Eoyang, G., E. Olson, G. Kennedy. *Complexity 101: Concepts and Tools for OD Practitioners.* Unpublished manuscript. p. 6.)

Groups that meet together and think together begin to learn each other's lingo. But what about encouraging an emerging group to create a subsystem of its own language and a cache of its own metaphors to help it move from an emerging organization to a stage of self-organization?

An emerging organization is often working to define itself and develop a sense of cohesion to achieve a specific goal within a specific time. The beginning of a new group's development, the creative or ideation period, most closely fits within the "random unpredictable" pattern, one of three patterns articulated in *Complexity 101* by Eoyang, Olson, and Kennedy.

"Random unpredictable" groups can evolve into complexly patterned groups as they calibrate the two variables of agreement and certainty and move into a self-organizing mode. A group cannot stay in the loose "random unpredictable" mode for very long without falling apart, yet it cannot maintain a self-organizing mode unless it attends to critical differences during its emergence stage. To speed through this period a little faster, rhyme "allows for humor, storytelling, and containment of anxieties" that release tension and urge action during this initial period of formation.

This article suggests that there is value for a newly-emerging group to build a vocabulary to monitor and "right" itself during its progression toward self-organization. Imagine this group as a collaboration of individuals who are not part of the same organization but represent a wide variety of different professional environments. Examples of such groups include appointed commissions, search committees, task forces, and boards of trustees or supervisors who meet infrequently and whose membership changes. Such groups move in nonlinear, iterative ways, with the ability to develop vocabularies to communicate through "shortcut phrases," which group members understand and respond to. Nonsense rhymes and children's stories provide possible shortcuts.

Rhymes and stories are self-contained, dynamic systems that provide paradoxes to illustrate poles of a spectrum between rigidity and boundlessness, with levels of permeability between. One good example of how polarity can be used to get us off the dime toward action is the poem "Alice," by Shel Silverstein, referring to Lewis Carroll's *Alice's Adventures in Wonderland:*

> She drank from a bottle called DRINK ME
>
> And up she grew so tall,
>
> She ate from a plate called TASTE ME,
>
> And down she shrank so small.

And so she changed, while other folks

Never tried nothin' at all.

One way to speed up the process of group commitment to change and to smooth a pathway for celebration, cohesion, and commonality within a group is to develop some common catch phrases, linguistic short cuts, that bring the group together and, in the process, provide a light touch and release of tension through humor. How better to accomplish the goals of tension release and progress than to utilize nonsensical rhyme, and children's stories and games? These rhymes and games have a certain level of simplicity to them, even though in many ways they reflect the complexity of working coherently with others to accomplish certain goals. Most of us are familiar with nonsensical rhyme. Many of us were exposed to such rhymes in our childhoods or as adults reading to children. Rhymes are intuitive, with sounds that ebb and flow as in nature because of their cadence. They often exhibit thought that is illogical to adults. The commonality of a child's pleasure in silly language is universal. Since such phrases do not reside in any one particular frame of reference, and since there is an inherent humor in nonsense, they already have attributes that release energy rather than constrain it. Why is nonsense so critical to emerging organizations and groups? In part, because it is the opposite of common sense, and common sense usually arises from individual behaviors in contexts outside the group. Nonsense allows for the dynamic process of a group defining a toolbox of catch phrases for itself.

Rhymes are useful societal teaching tools. They define appropriate behavior, sometimes by paradoxically illustrating quirks—behaviors at the margins—that emphasize difference. Examples of rhymes familiar to some of us from

Mother Goose are those about individuals such as Little Bo Peep and Little Boy Blue, who are careless with the care of their sheep; Jack Sprat (and his wife) and Jack and Jill— couples with skills that complement each other; and Old Mother Hubbard, a woman whose dog eventually gets the upper hand.

Other types of rhymes are more about groups than individuals and are called cumulative rhymes. Cumulative rhymes can be defined as those rhymes where actions logically and randomly pile upon each other. In these rhymes, the action follows a circuitous route to reach its goal. But just as water seeks the simplest, yet often the most complex route to fall into a level pool, rhymes seek the simplest way to communicate how complexity drives even the most simple action. Examples of goal statements are these: performing a service for others ("The Little Red Hen"), getting a stick to punish a recalcitrant animal or child ("The Old Woman and the Pig," or an Algerian version about feeding a child, or an Indian version that seeks to punish a crow for eating corn), paying for an animal (the Seder song "Two Zuzim"), or a Swahili rhyme that looks for who caused a tree to fall on a man (a slain deer swallowed a fly). These cumulative rhymes are the most useful in working with groups because they illustrate difference, document the building of a group's own history, and show how logical action is not reliable, predictable, or sometimes desirable.

A children's cumulative rhyme that can help a group focus on its emergent state is "The House That Jack Built." (The complete poem is provided at the end of this article.) How does this rhyme help to build a shared set of linguistic and behavioral codes for a group? First, it demonstrates how order emerges circuitously rather than hierarchically; second, it shows that all actions have a history that runs parallel to the immediate actions of the emergent group; and third, it demonstrates in a humorous way that a motley crew of participants, rather than the expected panel of experts, often comprises a set of critical builders and contributors to an emergent structure. All three attributes are evident in "The House That Jack Built." Both the rhyme and emerging organization share a sense of the interrelatedness of actions. Group participants recognize that what occurs is neither good nor bad but rather necessary to the consolidation of the internal dynamics of the group.

A Method for Introducing Nonsense

When a facilitator introduces nonsense rhymes as a theme for a series of group activities, he or she levels the playing field since such an introduction allows participants to detach from their professional moorings by losing the protective skin of their familiar and comfortable professional language. They move into an environment where they are expected to contribute and participate as equals and to help to create a vocabulary of catch phrases shared by the emergent group in their desire to develop the easiest means of communication.

The first group activity is to look at logical and illogical behavior of individuals and emerging groups. The facilitator asks if members of the group are familiar with "The House That Jack Built." After reading the cumulative rhyme, she asks how each person responds to it. Posting responses for all to see, the facilitator then points out how the rhyme includes a motley crew of people and animals, loosely connected, but all contributing to some ultimate goal related to the building of Jack's house.

To provide practice for the group, the facilitator then introduces a second but similar activity using the rhyme "The Old Woman and the Pig," which resembles the cumulative nature of "Jack," again asking for some ideas about what is going on. After the second set of responses is posted, the group members begin to talk about the lack of logic but at the same time the commonality of purpose of the players in the rhyme.

The "Old Mother Hubbard" story, familiar to many, is read as a third and final piece in this triad of cumulative rhymes. Participants are asked about the point of the poem. In considering the three rhymes, the group sees how actions accumulate and goals are expressed in nonsensical terms. Somehow goals are achieved in the rhymes: a dog is fed, a pig jumps over the wall, and a meal is eaten. As the group progresses, the catch phrases "it's like the house that Jack built," "it's like the old woman and the pig," it's like Old Mother Hubbard" provide shortcuts to providing a metaphor for the circuitous nature of group participation as well as group process. Nonsense becomes a metaphor for group thinking and group action.

As an interlude between the first and second sessions, or during the same session if necessary, the facilitator asks members of the group to access the web or to look through books or sheaves of rhymes and stories to find examples of rhymes that appeal to them and appear related to group development. These selected pieces become the basis of the group's often humorous discussion of logical and illogical behaviors of individuals and groups. The facilitator makes certain that the discussion focuses on how groups face emergence in order to expose the differences and uncertainties that are part of that path.

An additional exercise helps to focus on how to consider the progress of the group's emergence as being under-constrained or over-constrained. The group is asked to consider examples of polarities. Once the process begins, the suggestions cascade. "The Three Bears" story frequently emerges as one that contains polarities. As a group considers the elasticity of their framework ("their container") they size their frame for the process at hand. On a simple level, papa bear and mama bear represent the polarities of too hot/too cold, too hard/too soft, too big/too small versus the center "baby bear" point of just right. As emerging organizations and groups strive for the center point with the right level of elasticity, catch phrases such as "it's a little too hot in here" or "someone's been sitting in my chair" sends an electrical current through the group as members reflect together on the fit of the frame to the work at hand.

"The Three Little Pigs" and "Little Red Riding Hood" provide a different type of catch phrase. Instead of a set of poles with a center point as in "The Three Bears," these tales reveal a runaway train moving too fast down the track with a wreck in the offing. The straw and mud houses are too weak; only the better planned and executed house of brick will stand against the external forces or "wolf" that threatens it. The heat-absorbing brick kiln or incubator provides the needed planning time away from externalities — such as the wolf at the door. Just as everything in the "Three Little Pigs" indicates structures that are too weak, "Little Red Riding Hood" indicates forces that are too big. The wolf is again the symbol of externalities and everything about him is out of proportion (big eyes, big ears, and the final blow — big teeth).

As the group develops its own anthology and vocabulary, it gains strength and momentum, using humor to release tension along the way as a steam engine releases the energy that drives it. With this minimal level of preparation, groups can design this exercise any number of ways and times on an as-needed basis when the group determines that external forces threaten, logic prevails, or progress toward self organization is ebbing. Possibilities are endless — especially since the sources of rhymes and stories are not bounded by one language or one culture — and they are universal.

What follows are some examples from participants who selected a catch phrase to illustrate how the group might develop its vocabulary over time.

- By the end of "The House that Jack Built," I feel comfortable with the nonlinear route of our group's path and how the process is not causal but random. In the group, if I say "Jack's house," I mean that the current state of the group is dependent on all that has gone before — the group's history. We are not recreating ourselves each time we tackle a new problem.

- When I say "The old lady who lived in a shoe doesn't know what to do," I am saying that the group trying to remain organized is not necessarily the most important goal. Chaos brings the reward of the unexpected, and not knowing what to do is not so bad.

- When I say, "The dish ran away with the spoon," I mean that sometimes something else becomes a powerful attractor to a member of our group, and we just need to let that person go.

- When I say, "Little Jack Horner is in his corner," I mean that I miss his contributions. Somewhere we lost him and we need to reengage him.

- "1, 2, Buckle my shoe" means to me that we are in a repetitious cycle and going nowhere.

- When I say "Yankee Doodle" I mean that what something is and what we call it are quite different. (The rhyme reads, "Yankee Doodle stuck a feather in his hat and called it macaroni.")

- "They went to sea in a sieve" means to me that we need to make a decision fast. (The Edward Lear poem goes "Far and few, far and few, are the lands where the Jumblies live; their heads are green, and their hands are blue, and they went to sea in a sieve.")

- "This bed's too soft" means to me that our group needs to tighten up. Similarly, "This chair's too small" could mean that the group is overly constrained.

- "Painting the roses red" means to me that we are trying to make things into something else. (This Lewis Carroll phrase is from a description of the playing cards painting the white roses red, since they had planted the wrong color and the Queen of Hearts would likely be angry.)

- "Wouldn't that be grand!" means to me that we should tackle what is before us instead of the grandness we wish for. (The phrase is from Lewis Carroll: "The Walrus and the Carpenter were walking close at hand; they wept like anything to see such quantities of sand—'If this were only cleared away,' they said, 'it would be grand!'")

- "Rub-a-dub-dub, three men in a tub" inspires me to say that we are in this together and sometimes we need to shift to maintain balance."

The last exercise that often helps groups progress is focused on children's games, such as card games and playground games. These games illustrate some level of competitiveness. "Musical Chairs," seemingly an innocuous game, actually teaches the expectation of being left out, while "Ring Around the Rosy" indicates the expectation that everyone should get with the program. The card games "Go Fish" and "Crazy Eights" promote the collections of similarities, while "War" is confrontational at every turn of the card and plays on differences.

- "Go Fish" means to me that I don't have what you need, but take a chance and choose from what's left in the middle pile.

- "Ring Around the Rosy...we all fall down" means to me that competition can become cooperation if everyone takes a chance and participates.

- "Pop Goes the Weasel" means to me that surprises happen, even when we think the music is so methodical.

- "Musical chairs" means that if any one of us removes a place or discounts a participant, some one of us will be left out.

This article has proposed that ways to develop group identity and to dissipate barriers are to develop a common, albeit nonsensical, language to serve as a release rather than a constraint—even if for a short period. Some groups may balk at defining a set of catch phrases. However, recalibration of communication may save them time and may streamline their progress and definitely will infuse their processes with humor. Self-organizing suggests that resonance among a collection of people arises at their intersections rather than within each person. The assumption is that these intersections are dynamic, flexible, and malleable, as is language.

By serendipitously building up schemas and knocking them over with rhymes, as children do with their blocks by a seemingly random action, the desire to create a single, perfect design evaporates and allows for continual emergence and reemergence of an order that makes sense for a particular, emerging group. This emergence is not of the type where a caterpillar transforms into a butterfly after a stay in a cocoon; rather, it is the morphing of a landscape of group thought, such that adjustments throughout the system occur randomly, and shocks to a system are not reduced to logic. Order follows rather than leads. The hope is that developing networks, with their reinforced interlace, have the strength of a shared pattern and the stickiness of a spider's web. Stickiness can arise through the web of language. Such a web becomes a net loosely but flexibly offering a means to move from the loosely connected ends toward the more tightly woven center of the web matrix. Such movement resembles the movement of emerging groups from random to self-organizing states.

As Reuben McDaniel states, "Uncertainty is fundamental in the world, and you can't resolve uncertainty through more information or more processing of information." Processing nonsensical language allows a group to participate in illogical, circuitous thinking, and thereby make speedier headway toward defining and redefining a common goal during a period of emergence. Nonsense rhymes embrace a system by enhancing interactivity and sparking different synapses that organizational languages often pass by.

This is the House that Jack Built

This is the House that Jack Built.

This is the malt that lay in the house that Jack built.

This is the rat that ate the malt that lay in the house that Jack built.

This is the cat that killed the rat that ate the malt that lay in the house that Jack built.

This is the dog that worried the cat that killed the rat that ate the malt that lay in the house that Jack built.

This is the cow with the crumpled horn that tossed the dog that worried the cat that killed the rat that ate the malt that lay in the house that Jack built.

This is the maiden all forlorn that milked the cow with the crumpled horn that tossed the dog that worried the cat that killed the rat that ate the malt that lay in the house that Jack built.

This is the man all tattered and torn that kissed the maiden all forlorn that milked the cow with the crumpled horn that tossed the dog that worried the cat that killed the rat that ate the malt that lay in the house that Jack built.

This is the priest all shaven and shorn that married the man all tattered and torn that kissed the maiden all forlorn that milked the cow with the crumpled horn that tossed the dog that worried the cat that killed the rat that ate the malt that lay in the house that Jack built.

This is the cock that crowed in the morn that waked the priest all shaven and shorn that married the man all tattered and torn that kissed the maiden all forlorn that milked the cow with the crumpled horn that tossed the dog that worried the cat that killed the rat that ate the malt that lay in the house that Jack built.

This is the farmer sowing the corn that kept the cock that crowed in the morn that waked the priest all shaven and shorn that married the man all tattered and torn that kissed the maiden all forlorn that milked the cow with the crumpled horn that tossed the dog that worried the cat that killed the rat that ate the malt that lay in the house that Jack built.

Gayle Byock

Gayle's nonlinear career has taken her from studying Latin and writing poetry; through teaching at the junior high school, high school, community college, college, and university levels; to administrating everything from projects to policy development in the University of California, Los Angeles Chancellor's Office. She has spent 20 years at UCLA in many wonderful roles that required her to learn the fundamentals of complexity science and organizational development. She helped to design and create emerging institutes, offices, and a school within the university structure.

As Director Of Higher Education Relationships and in response to a reconsideration of the California Master Plan of Higher Education in the 1980s, Gayle developed the Transfer Alliance Program that continues to be a model of a comprehensive relationship between about thirty California community colleges and the university. In the 1990s she worked to incorporate ethnicity and gender issues into mainstream courses and, later, as Assistant Dean, she helped to found the School of Public Policy and Social Research, the first

UCLA professional school in 30 years. As Assistant Vice Chancellor of Research, she worked until 2001 to improve the research infrastructure of the campus by facilitating multidisciplinary teams of faculty from the eleven professional schools and the College of Letters and Science as well as by initiating more customer-focused Offices of Contracts and Grants and Technology Transfer. In 2001, Gayle began designing and implementing models of sustainable, long-term research and learning relationship among six Los Angeles communities of need and many students, faculty, and administrators across the campus.

In addition to campus activities, Gayle has worked with international, national and state initiatives to promote a wide variety of uses of technology in health, multimedia, urban planning, the arts and the sciences. She has developed a concept called The Higher Education Trust as a means to deliver comprehensive, collaborative partnerships between colleges and universities and communities and schools. With corporations and institutes she has worked on issues from the delivery of distance learning and the use of the Internet around the globe to local economic development. Most recently, Gayle has moved into activities that combine her interests and experience in the delivery of education and health care to groups who lack access to both. Gayle invites questions or comments via email at gaylebyock@yahoo.com.

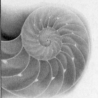

WHAT DOES IT REALLY TAKE TO BRING A GROUP TOGETHER INTO COORDINATED ACTION? ONCE THE GROUP IS FORMED, HOW DOES IT SUSTAIN ENERGY AND FOCUS? HOW DOES A LEADER MAINTAIN INDIVIDUAL SATISFACTION WHILE CONSTRUCTING SUFFICIENT CONSENSUS FOR ACTION? NEAL KAUFMAN HAS LIVED THE ANSWERS TO THESE QUESTIONS. AS A COMMUNITY LEADER, PHYSICIAN, AND EXECUTIVE MANAGER, NEAL HAS CONFRONTED SOME VERY DIFFICULT GROUP DYNAMICS. THE TIPS HE PROVIDES HERE ARE GLEANED FROM THOSE EXPERIENCES AND A PROFOUND UNDERSTANDING OF COMPLEX DYNAMICS OF HUMAN SYSTEMS.

Sustaining Results and the Relationships on Which They are Built

By Neal Kaufman, M.D., M.P.H.

All of us have struggled to create that which should be sustained and to sustain what has been created. To develop, implement, and sustain a successful program requires a lot of wisdom, hard work, perseverance, and some luck.

For most of my career I have been a "horizontalist" in a vertical world...a vertical world of increasing specialization, of increasing attempts to solve problems by dividing the components into ever smaller parts. My horizontalist approach of integrating and coordinating services and supports lacked a coherent and theoretical basis. In the spirit of complexity, I randomly came upon the science of complex adaptive systems when I heard a talk by an expert in complexity science. I instantly recognized the inherent wisdom of the theoretical framework and ever since, my worlds have begun to make sense.

As a creator of some successful and some not so successful health programs, I certainly have no corner on wisdom, but I have had some great teachers who have taught me the value of **F*R*I*E*N*D*S***. Here are some of the lessons I have learned and my own personal guides for improving health. I hope you find them helpful.

Friendships: Create positive relationships between individuals and between members of organizations.

Results: Distribute rewards based on results.

Information: Assure the free flow of timely and accurate data, information, knowledge, and wisdom.

Emergence: Encourage new and innovative ideas and practices through the creative energies of individuals.

Nurturing: Assure everyone is loved, nurtured, safe, and intellectually stimulated.

Dollars: Provide easy access to adequate resources for everyone.

Strong Communities: Strengthen every community and all families.

More on Each

Friendships: Create positive relationships between individuals and between members of organizations.

Have Friends — and Lots of Them
Developing friends, allies, and collaborators based on mutual respect and recognition of each person's strengths early in a project can help to overcome most barriers. Good relationships remain productive long after the end of the circumstances under which they were started. Try to create safe, protected ways for all participants to support open, honest, and creative reflections on what's happening and what's being learned.

Network with Everyone
Networks provide support while also triggering innovative approaches that build upon what is already in existence. This is especially true if the networks are made up of people with diverse backgrounds, ideas, experiences and approaches. A good network contains a balance of individuals who are:

- Verticalists (those who specialize in relevant areas)

- Horizontalists (those who synthesize from across many focused areas)

- Connectors (those who are linked to a variety of people)

- Sales people (those who can explain ideas and convince others).

Networks also increase adaptability when trying to successfully cope with the surprises—both good and bad—that always seem to happen. Don't require collaborators to meet an artificially high standard for administrative competence. Just the presence and support of others can move an agenda along in ways that are not always obvious (e.g., relationships to key decision makers, joining one agenda to another).

Results: Distribute rewards based on results.

Give Credit

You can accomplish more if you don't care who gets the credit, but be sure to give credit when credit is due.

Focus on the results the group is seeking and create a team that rewards people, organizations, and systems for the outcomes they obtain. Identifying hoped-for outcomes in advance, and not the details of the process to get there, allows creative solutions to emerge. Be sure to break down results into small attainable outcomes so you don't have to wait till the final result is reached before a reward is given. Everyone needs to recognize that despite best efforts and good thinking, hoped-for results may not be achieved. Rewards should go to people who try new things, create networks/relationships, and work to establish conditions to foster healthier communities. While recognizing small actions can lead to major and often unpredictable changes, try to develop ways to reward collaborators for the proportion of the outcome for which they are responsible while supporting and recognizing the work of the whole.

Plan for Success, Learn from Failures

Successful failures are critical sources of learning. If they are not celebrated, people will hide them and not do constructive evaluations. Anyone who makes a mistake has done a favor to the organization if a lesson can be learned from the mistake. This requires a very safe and supportive environment where such matters can be discussed openly without threatening individuals or relationships. Don't get upset about the time it takes to implement change. If something is important, don't give up; keep trying to find better ways to make it happen.

Learn to Say No—Gently

In the process of balancing creativity with practicality, learn to distinguish between those requests that deserve preserving from those that should be stopped or changed. Sometimes an early rejection is a favor that prevents an abject failure.

Reject the Conspiracy of Hyperbole

A conspiracy of hyperbole occurs when organizations seek funds, promise everything and funding agencies tell their governing bodies the world will become a perfect place because of their wise funding decisions. Be honest with yourself and the funding source regarding the potential for change and the problems you expect to encounter. This will build real trust and credibility.

Make Things Real

Provide an opportunity for those making important decisions to experience the group's mission and activities. Let them meet the people being served, witness the needs, see the change, and feel rewarded by having contributed to something valuable.

Information: Assure the free flow of timely and accurate data, information, knowledge, and wisdom.

Provide Information
Assure the free flow of timely and accurate:

- Data — discrete objective facts

- Information — data with meaning

- Knowledge — framework for evaluating information and new experiences

- Wisdom — insight/intuitive knowing

Communicate to build trust and maintain interest while recognizing many things are not as they might appear, especially because of the range of interpretations possible from similar data. Telling the hard truths and the bad news is what makes the good news credible.

Keep Things Simple
Most successes occur when the concepts are simplified so people can understand them. Failure often occurs when issues, suggestions, or programs are too complicated. Strive to make everything you do understandable to the least experienced person in the system, including the consumer. One way to be sure things are understandable to a wide audience is to have diversity among the members of the team.

Spread Innovation Gradually
Help nurture the adoption of innovations by working with a small number of well-connected early adopters. Once successful, use them and their networks to facilitate further spread of the innovation leading to universal acceptance.

Emergence: Encourage emergence of new and innovative ideas and practices through the creative energies of individuals.

Plant Seedlings and Watch What Grows

Try something different, encourage unusual approaches to solving problems, consciously work outside conventional arenas, and incorporate a diversity of voices and approaches in all you do. Be aware of the successes around you by discovering useful patterns of behaviors leading to innovation. Be alert for the promising seeds of an idea that arrive unexpectedly, not according to any schedule and often at times when things are feeling uncomfortable. By trying many small changes simultaneously rather than one large change, you are more likely to stumble on a good solution and stimulate unforeseeable ripple effects leading to sustainable innovations. When you discover something that works, do more of it.

Determine Good-enough Processes

While focusing on outcomes, also remember processes determine outcomes. Don't create inflexible processes or systems. Rather, allow continuous improvements to emerge through the creative ideas of all participants.

Balance Vision with Practicality

While it is important to have a big picture and a grand vision, incremental improvements are usually the most successful way to sustain changes. The most successful approaches nurture that balance over time, leading to innovative and sustainable changes. While some seek opportunities, the more successful seek goals. Your vision should be based not on what funding is available, but rather on the changes you want to see.

Lead Humbly

Don't assume leaders can single-handedly plan and implement changes. Even when key decision-makers agree to make something happen, there is no guarantee it will occur. Not only can priorities change, but no leader can affect more than 15–20 percent of the things around him or her.

<u>N</u>urturing: Assure everyone is loved, nurtured, safe, and intellectually stimulated.

Nurture Team Members

How people are treated and supported is reflected in the ways they treat others. The true spirit of collaboration is not about assembling a team to implement your ideas, but to create a true working group that becomes self-directing and self-nourishing. Look for ways to keep members of the team fulfilled and feeling good about themselves and their roles. When trying to bring about change, it is often difficult to see the benefits — frustration and discouragement are all too frequent. Helping team members experience things that are going well can go a long way toward personal satisfaction and improved morale. After all, people are the most important part of any project.

Feed People's Minds and Stomachs

Nutrition and nurturing are linked from earliest infancy when we were loved and fed by our mothers (and fathers). We intuitively feel comforted by food, and it helps to enhance relationships and foster partnerships. Never ignore a chance to break bread with your collaborators and with those who might not agree with you. Providing food at group gatherings will help cement the bonds of friendship and collaboration.

Dollars: Provide easy access to adequate resources for everyone.

Sustain through Connections
Make connections with existing approaches and programs to create a lattice-like safety network to support your goals. Building on existing connections to close gaps (rather than creating completely new solutions) will provide strong scaffolding for sustainability. The strongest connections are those in which all participants believe everyone wins if anyone wins, and everyone loses if anyone loses. Even if one part of the network is not successful, the strength of the connections will sustain the results.

Create What Should be Sustained and Sustain What Should be Created
While it is sometimes very natural to believe programs or organizations should be sustained for their own sake, we should aim to sustain visions, partners, and outcomes. This occurs when we sustain core ideas, values and the beliefs behind the work; relationships and the connections they maintain; management strengths and leadership; collective goals and commitment; increased capacity of individuals, families, organizations, and the community.

Choose Interventions Strategically to Sustain Results
When trying to plan for the future, first try to identify the individual, institutional, and/or system-wide changes (e.g., attitudes, policies and procedures) which will be necessary to sustain your hoped-for goals. Target your efforts toward the administrative enhancements, specific program/services, and policy actions which will document the strengths and weakness of the specific approaches taken and the long-term

policy changes necessary to dispense the innovation widely and to sustain the changes.

Survive after Funding Ends

Creating a project which raises people's expectations and having it become successful, only to have it collapse when initial funding is exhausted can do more harm than good. Have a real strategy for sustainability from the beginning of the project, and expect to re-think it several times during the life of the project. Even though the original plans will probably not be followed at the end, attention to sustainability from the start will help in crafting a viable strategy.

Self-Promote for Sustainability

From the beginning of a project supported by a foundation or other entity, be sure to have the group capitalize on the stamp of approval the support affords and to share the glory with collaborators. Don't be modest. Shamelessly capitalize on the good will and potential benefits of being selected in a highly competitive process. This self-promotion is really in the best interest of your program.

Strong Communities: Strengthen every community and all families.

Improve Health Holistically

Individuals are only as healthy as the families in which they live, and families are only as healthy as the communities in which they reside. Always consider each person in the context of his or her family and community. Communities need healthy environments, organizations, and associations that nurture everyone. Be sure to help develop the networks of support and services so essential for a healthy community. Communities in turn are nurtured by a society that recognizes the importance of every individual, acknowledges the inter-connections of all individuals, and provides the support necessary for each person to achieve his or her potential. Create ways for individuals and organizations to advocate effectively on behalf of healthy individuals, families, and communities.

Create Links

Link community nests of support, medical homes, systems for early care and lifelong learning, and centers for education and quality.

Four segments of society need to be supported to create sustainable and effective approaches to improving the health of a population:

- <u>Community nests of support</u> (e.g., formal and informal community support networks, and social services agencies) provide essential health, educational and human services.

- <u>Medical homes</u>, based in physicians' offices and clinics, assure global health needs of a person are meet by being part of networks of integrated services.

- <u>Systems for Early Care and Lifelong Learning</u> (e.g., childcare, preschools, schools, adult education programs) provide critical learning opportunities and connections.

- <u>Centers for Education and Quality</u> (e.g., academic medical centers, universities, and colleges) provide opportunities for direct services, professional training, and research.

It is especially critical that these sites link to each other through collaborative relationships and joint projects.

FRIENDS in Action: an Example from the Field

Several years ago, I worked with a health clinic to improve the quality of the medical care and customer service provided to children and their families in the context of house-staff education. Over a one-year period, the staff and providers went through an extensive and time-consuming process of getting information from everyone who worked in the clinic to create detailed operational flowcharts. These diagrams painstakingly documented the ways these individuals thought things were being done and were used to develop consensus about the new way things should be done to improve the clinic's function. Unfortunately, little improved. Even with the best intentions, the clinic was still having problems. From what I know now about complexity science, I'm not surprised they weren't successful.

After many years with minimal improvement, the clinic staff were ready for a new way. It was decided to use some of the principles of complexity science to guide the activities. Since the clinic is part of a larger facility, the staff first needed to redesign their relationship to the facility leadership group. In the past, the facility leadership group made all policies and developed all procedures, expecting the clinic staff to implement them. The facility leadership group agreed to redefine their role: to set the vision; help define overall goals; and enable things to happen by supporting the staff and removing barriers outside of the staff's control.

The facility leadership team first set out a "good-enough" but lofty vision for the clinic: "The Health Clinic will be nationally recognized as a premier patient care and resident teaching center." The staff set the specific results they wanted to see, such as decreased patient time in registration, decreased total patient visit time, decreased time waiting on the phone;

increased patient, parent and physician satisfaction; and improved relationships between the doctors and nurses. Staff decided how to accomplish these goals by setting their own guidelines. Two strategies used were nonhierarchical decision-making and rapid-cycle improvement.

The team implemented new approaches, evaluated their usefulness, and modified approaches according to the results. For example, hospital administration mandated no overtime for clinic staff. The facility leadership team passed on this information and the clinic staff developed specific practices, which led to the elimination of overtime. They used a similar methodology to help staff learn how to get authorization for referrals. One non-clinic staff member figured out how to work successfully with government programs and the team wanted to share her wisdom with the clinic staff. Instead of scheduling formal in-service education programs or creating formal policies, the skilled person informally talked with the clinic staff to help them learn how to problem-solve on their own. These informal discussions led to the creation of "good-enough" guidelines on obtaining authorizations. The clinic made such notable progress that six months later it received the Institution's Nursing Unit of the Year Award for Innovation and Improvement in the Delivery of Patient Care; the first time an outpatient clinic had ever won this award.

While this example doesn't address all of the issues raised by FRIENDS, I hope it helps you to see that using these principles can lead to real changes in everyday activities.

Neal Kaufman, M.D., M.P.H.

Neal Kaufman, M.D., M.P.H., is Director of the Division of Primary Care Pediatrics and holder of the Guess?/Fashion Industries Guild Chair in Community Child Health at Cedars-Sinai Medical Center. In addition, he is Professor of Pediatrics and Public Health at the University of California, Los Angeles (UCLA), Schools of Medicine and Public Health, and Co-Director of the UCLA Center for Healthier Children, Families and Communities.

Dr. Kaufman is also a commissioner on the Los Angeles County Children and Families First Commission, a large government-based, grant-making foundation with the goal of improving the well-being of children by their fifth birthday.

Dr. Kaufman has been a leader in local, state, and national efforts to improve the health of children, particularly those who are low income and at high risk. He is an expert in a wide range of areas including delivery of healthcare to high risk and vulnerable women and children, health advocacy for women, children and families, healthcare for abused and neglected children and adolescents, and house staff education in primary care. He advises a number of local, state, and national legislators on methods to improve the health of children, families, and communities.

Dr. Kaufman has been a member of the Academy of Pediatrics' national Committee on Early Childhood, Adoption and Dependency, as well as the American Public Health Association's Task Force on Child Health, National March of Dimes Birth Defects Foundation's Office of Volunteers, and several national and local professional societies. He received his bachelor's degree from Northwestern University and his medical degree from The Chicago Medical School. He completed pediatric training at Childrens Hospital Los Angeles and public health training at UCLA.

LESLIE PATTERSON AND CAROL WICKSTROM BELIEVE DEEPLY THAT SHARED INQUIRY IS THE PATH TO LEARNING. THEY USE THIS CONVICTION, THEIR EXPERIENCE AS MASTER TEACHERS, AND THEIR UNDERSTANDING OF HUMAN SYSTEMS DYNAMICS TO ESTABLISH A PROFESSIONAL DEVELOPMENT NETWORK OF MIDDLE SCHOOL TEACHERS. HERE THEY DESCRIBE THE CONDITIONS THE GROUP SET FOR ITS OWN SELF-ORGANIZING, HOW THE STRUCTURES AND FUNCTIONS OF THE NETWORK RESPONDED, AND HOW THE EMERGING NETWORK SUPPORTS SHARED INQUIRY AMONG STUDENTS, FACULTY, AND ADMINISTRATION.

MIDDLE SCHOOL TEACHERS ON THE CUTTING EDGE OF LITERACY INSTRUCTION

By Leslie Patterson, Ph.D. and Carol Wickstrom, Ph.D.

With contributions by Debbie Boatright, Jody Carter, Sonja Edwards, Randy Freeman, Mollie Furrh, Lisa Heiens, Pam Holland, Julie Keith, Elizabeth Luttmer, and Linda Whiddon

Bureaucratic solutions to problems of practice will always fail because effective teaching is not routine, students are not passive, and questions of practice are not simple, predictable or standardized. Consequently, instructional decisions cannot be formulated on high then packaged and handed down to teachers. (Darling-Hammond, 1997, p. 67)

Research findings point to the compelling (and not surprising) conclusion that thoughtful teachers make the difference for student learning. The most effective schools have teachers who are mindful decision-makers—teachers who have learned to watch their students carefully and draw both on their classroom experience and on published research (Allington, 2002; Carlson & Apple, 1998; Freire, 1998; Patterson & Mallow, 2001; Taylor, Pearson, Clark, and Walpole, 1999; Wickstrom & Curtis, 2002). They respond in unique ways to each student. They know that, just as no two learners are alike, no two teaching decisions can be the same.

Unfortunately, professional development initiatives for teachers typically focus on one-size-fits-all techniques, rather than thoughtful decision-making. As the opening quote points out, "questions of practice are not simple, predictable or standardized," and these formulaic approaches will not work. This point is particularly timely in light of the 2001 "No Child Left Behind Act" mandate for "scientifically" proven programs, a mandate which can be interpreted as endorsing commercial programs, rather than encouraging professionals to make decisions that respond to local needs.

This chapter describes an alternative approach in a medium-sized middle school in a small town in south-central United States. The school's principal and faculty are currently engaged in a school-wide reform effort, with particular attention to reading instruction. The teachers, the principal, the school improvement facilitator, and two university professors are using "collaborative conversations" (Hollingsworth, 1994) to refine their teaching decisions and to document how their students respond. This article is the beginning of their story.

The Conceptual Framework

Carol and Leslie, the university professors who were invited to lead this professional development effort, began with the assumption that the students, teachers, and staff comprise a complex network of massively entangled social systems. We used concepts from the CDE Model of self-organizing systems delineated by Glenda Eoyang (Eoyang, 2001) to help the work self-organize into a coherent, campus-wide approach to reading/language arts instruction. The goal was to engage the teachers in an inquiry process to refine and modify what was already working for their students, to set conditions that would encourage each teacher to learn what published research might contribute, and to develop a set of approaches for this context, for these students.

Historically, policy-makers and administrators have assumed a factory metaphor for schooling that says the world is linear, predictable, and controllable. This approach assumes components work together in mechanical ways and problems are solved by taking things apart, repairing the pieces, and re-assembling them. This perspective inspires high-stakes accountability schemes and curricular mandates. It also inspires reductionist school reform models, centralized decision-making, and the de-professionalization of teachers.

Complexity science, on the other hand, suggests that much of the world is comprised of interconnected complex adaptive systems — groups of agents that join together for common purposes, purposes related to sustaining the system (Eoyang, 1997; Goldstein, 1994; Olson & Eoyang, 2001, Lissack & Roos, 1999; Stacey, 2001; Stewart & Cohen, 1999; Waldrop, 1992). These systems are organic; they grow and mature. When applied to schooling and, more specifically, when applied to campus-based reform and professional development, this perspective can make quite a difference.

To see what a difference this perspective can make, consider the following assumptions about how complex adaptive systems within schools work. These assumptions are based on Eoyang's delineation of the CDE Model of self-organizing systems. (Eoyang, 2001):

- We cannot control or predict what will happen, although we can sometimes recognize patterns or trends, even when things at first appear random or disconnected.

- We often see similar dynamics across various "scales" in the system — the individual, the classroom, the faculty, the campus, the district, the community, etc.

- Self-organizing systems are massively entangled, interconnected, and interdependent.

- These systems are always changing, and histories (of the parts and the whole) are critically meaningful.

- At each scale, complex adaptive systems manifest three conditions: container, difference, and transformative exchanges.

- When forces within or outside the system exert sufficient pressure, system-wide patterns emerge to allow the system to adapt and remain viable, and we say the system self-organizes.

- These emergent patterns — the new whole — is inherently different from (not necessarily better) than a sum of the old parts. In schools, these emergent patterns may support student learning, but alternative patterns may emerge that interfere with student learning.

- To the extent that agents can influence the conditions of the system (container, difference, and transformative exchanges), they can influence the direction and character of self-organization.

These assumptions acknowledge the power of agents (students, parents, faculty, and administrators) to influence the system by learning more about what is happening and how to change what is not working. This work can be thought of as a spiraling and recursive inquiry cycle through which teachers ask and answer three questions, revisiting each question again and again as the system changes or as the agents' understandings of the system changes:

- What's happening?
- So what does it mean?
- Now what shall we do about it?

These questions provide a lens to examine Eoyang's conditions of self-organizing systems: container, difference, and transformative exchanges.

Container, Difference, and Transformative Exchanges

The "container" of a self-organizing system refers to whatever provides its coherence, whatever makes this system different from its context. Containers can be signified by labels (names, titles, ethnicities, gender, mottoes, etc.) or by place (geographical locations, physical spaces, etc.) or by shared work (objectives, missions, worldviews, perspectives, methods, etc.). All of these types of containers appear in school systems, among teachers, and within classrooms, among students.

Difference across a self-organizing system is critical. If there are no significant differences, if the system is homogeneous, it will not change. It is static; some would call it a system in homeostasis. On the other hand, if there are so many differences that none stands out as critical, the system cannot self-organize or adapt. It will probably cease to be a "system" because there is no container—not enough similarities to hold the system together. For this reason, differences between and among teachers can be significant. Student strengths, ethnicities, and achievement levels can also point to significant differences.

Another way to think about difference is to think about where we are now and where we want to go. In that sense, curriculum standards and standardized test objectives point to differences that make a difference in a school improvement initiative. The consultants in this project tried to find out what these teachers perceived as the differences that made a difference to their students' literacy learning, and they tried to make those differences public and open to discussion—the focus of our collaborative inquiry.

Multiple opportunities to exchange information and energy are a final condition of self-organizing systems. In a nonhuman system, like an ecosystem, transformative exchanges most often involve the exchange of energy and information. In social systems, transformative exchanges involve the exchange of information or resources that support the system's work. Meetings, memos, e-mail, professional readings, conversations, lesson plans, budgets, expenditures for instructional materials—all these can serve as transformative exchanges.

The list of questions below was suggested by these three conditions—questions that teachers, administrators, and staff developers can use to trigger and sustain self-organizing systems to support school improvement. These are interdependent questions; the listing implies no priority; and this list is not meant to suggest a procedure or rigid protocol.

Questions to Sustain Self-organizing Teaching/Learning Systems

Who are We and What Are We About?
- Who are we?

- What are we about?

- What is our "work" together?

- What are our shared values?

- What are our shared goals?

What Differences Make a Difference to Our Work?
- What are the differences between what we see now and what we want to see?

- Which differences among us offer a potential for shared learning?

- Which differences among us are directly relevant to our work?

- Which differences among us are irrelevant to our work?

- Which differences among us have the potential for interfering with our work?

How Do We Teach and Learn across These Significant Differences?
- How often should we communicate with one another?

- How can we set up multiple exchanges between individuals and among groups?

- How can we ensure that these are two-way exchanges?

- How can we ensure that the content of these exchanges reinforces issues related to our system container and significant differences?

- How can we keep records of our exchanges, to make them accessible for individual and collaborative reflection and analysis?

- How do we ensure that we give and get value for value?

These questions can be used in various ways to trigger conversations, decisions, and actions that contribute to the work of the group. In the following discussion, we draw primarily on meeting notes and the website from the Decatur Middle School project to examine whether our understanding of these conditions is helping the group move toward self-organization.

Who Are We and What Are We About?

Decatur, Texas is a small town of just over 5,000 people, forty miles northwest of Fort Worth, Texas. Approximately half of these people are students in one of its five public schools. The ethnicity of students in Decatur schools is typical of many rural Texas towns, with about three-quarters of the students listed as white and almost a quarter Hispanic. Less than ten percent of the students are "limited-English proficient," and one-third of the students are "economically disadvantaged." The district has recently received $1.3 million for a three-year implementation of Accelerated Schools — a school-wide reform process. According to the district website, "The Accelerated Schools philosophy reinforces the District vision of providing the best education for each student by empowering teachers with campus decision-making opportunities and research-based teaching strategies facilitating learning." (http://www.decatur.esc11.net)

Accelerated Schools is an inquiry-based reform effort that encourages teachers and staff to participate in a collaborative inquiry and action cycle to provide school-wide support for student achievement (Hopfenberg, Levin, and Associates, 1993). At the Decatur Middle School campus, teachers targeted several areas. One was reading achievement/engagement among their seventh and eighth graders. These reading and language arts teachers wanted to build on the approaches that the elementary teachers in the district had begun using, but they didn't know much about those approaches. Consultants from a nearby university were called in to teach the teachers how to use those approaches.

In May, 2002, Leslie met with Linda, the principal, Lisa, and Debbie to talk about possibilities for a professional development project for middle school Reading/Language Arts teachers. It was decided that over the summer the teachers would read *I Read It, but I Don't Get It: Comprehension Strategies for Adolescent Readers* by Cris Tovani and Ellin Oliver Keene (2000) to prepare for monthly study group meetings in September.

In September, Carol joined me as a consultant on the project, and worked primarily with the history teachers. During the following fall and winter, she and I would meet with the teachers, principal, and Pam, the Accelerated Schools project coach/facilitator, on one Wednesday afternoon a month, from 1:30 to 3:30. Substitutes covered the teachers' classes. This discussion focuses on the work of the reading/language arts teachers.

In our September meeting, we talked about what we had learned from the book we had read over the summer and how everyone had begun using the ideas in his or her classroom. We pointed out that not many middle school teachers across the country had joined campus-wide efforts like this — that we were on the cutting edge as we applied these new approaches with middle school students. When we talked about what we wanted to call ourselves, Debbie suggested "The Bladerunners," and that's what we became.

To influence the system to move toward self-organizing learning, we made decisions that made our "container" explicit. The group's name, the book to be read, the meeting times and place, the planning group (principal and consultants), the inclusion of only reading/language arts and history teachers, the distinction between the instruction in elementary and middle schools, the decision to focus on a specific list of comprehension strategies — all these decisions helped define our group and our work. Those distinctions made this project, these teachers, and their work together somehow different from everything else going on at the campus. The teachers began talking to their colleagues and to district administrators about the "University of North Texas (UNT) Collaborative," and that is the label that has most clearly defined this container for them. Without such a container — this explicit shared identity or common work—we could not have moved forward toward any kind of systemic change or self-organization.

What Differences Make a Significant Difference to Our Students' Literacy?

In Texas public schools, the state curriculum standards (Texas Essential Knowledge and Skills, or TEKS) and the state-mandated criterion-referenced test (Test of Academic

Knowledge and Skills, or TAKS) point to mandated differences that make a difference to teachers and students. These teachers, however, did not want to focus narrowly on test preparation. Their students performed fairly well on these tests, so we looked for additional differences that would make a difference in the literacy lives of these students.

In the first meeting, the teachers asked for information about "guided reading." In the years since the first introduction of "guided reading" in the lower grades, these middle school teachers had noted that incoming 7th graders seemed to be more knowledgeable and enthusiastic readers. The teachers wanted to know more about how to build on this foundation to prepare students for high school and beyond. Their questions seemed to focus on "how to do" this instructional approach — the methodology and the classroom routine.

The book we read over the summer, however, did not name "guided reading" as a methodology that made a difference. Instead, it delineated reading strategies that proficient, independent readers use and explained how to encourage and support strategic reading. After discussing the book and thinking about their own students, the Bladerunners came up with their customized list of strategies — a list they could agree on as a focus for reading instruction across all their classes. These are the strategies, they decided, that would make a difference to their students:

- Connecting
- Questioning
- Inferring
- Monitoring and repairing understanding

- Determining what's important

- Synthesizing

- Visualizing

- Responding emotionally

By the second monthly meeting, the discussion had begun moving away from instructional methodology as the difference that makes a difference to focus on the students and how to engage the students in meaning-making.

The teachers invited a fifth grade teacher to our second meeting to show a video of her students. The video also actually showed fifth graders engaged in lively discussions about a book, clearly using the comprehension strategies on our list. The teacher talked about how she taught her students to participate in these discussions. At that point, we realized that what we wanted to learn about was not "guided reading," but how to encourage students to read critically and to participate enthusiastically in open-ended, student-led discussions.

Our discussion of that video triggered two discoveries. First, it showed us what we wanted students to learn to do. Second, it helped us see that we really were not as interested in instructional methods (like guided reading) as we were in students' independent use of these powerful comprehension strategies. For us, that became the difference that made the difference. It no longer seemed appropriate to identify one instructional approach or method for everyone. That was a significant difference that remained important throughout the year.

In November, at our third meeting, Mollie and the other English teachers voiced a concern about needing to spend more time on writing instruction than on the reading strategies that had been our focus to that point. That prompted us to acknowledge that these comprehension strategies also would support students' writing. When we decided to make a conscious shift to include both reading and writing strategies in our discussions, the English teachers became more engaged in the group inquiry. The difference between reading and writing instruction no longer made a difference.

In December, we decided to focus on one specific strategy— "connecting." We realized that when we talked about all the strategies at once, our conversations were abstract. When we focused on one strategy, we could cite particular student responses. We could talk specifically about what makes a "great connection." We developed a rubric to guide our assessment of students' connections in their reading and writing. It soon became clear that "connections" in reading are parallel to "elaboration" in writing. It was a small step from that insight to identifying what strategic elaboration would look like in student writing.

After only four meetings, we had made important progress in terms of the differences we saw as significant. We had moved from focusing on teaching methods to focusing on student engagement and strategy use. We had also moved from an abstract discussion of comprehension strategies to a specific focus on "connecting" as a powerful strategy. In addition, we had moved from a limited focus on reading to the more comprehensive focus on reading and writing as two ways to view strategic comprehension. That led to the recognition of how the instruction in "reading" class can build on what is going on in "English" class. It was not enough simply to identify an initial difference that made a difference, like a goal statement for the group. The continual search for more specific, more significant differences mediated our conversations and our discoveries. Looking for the differences that made the difference fueled our collaborative learning.

Within this progression, the work became more focused and more tied to doing, rather than just thinking or talking. The container shifted and became more focused, or "smaller." As the container shifted, different differences were clearly significant. As we articulated the differences within each emerging container, our dialogue provided a structure that allowed us to focus on even more relevant and significant differences. Our collaborative conversations, in this way, provided a dynamic scaffolding for our emerging insights and our new questions — our self-organizing understandings of strategic reading and writing.

How Are We Teaching and Learning Across those Significant Differences?

Our initial understanding of the CDE Model made it clear that we should institute a number of potentially transformational exchanges. First, we read published accounts of teachers' inquiries. Those common readings and our discussions provided the basis for our collaborative learning. The teachers, however, did not immediately use our monthly discussions as a forum for free-flowing dialogue. During the first meetings, the teachers seemed to expect that Carol and I would do most of the talking. Maybe everyone was expecting a "telling" model that is more typical of professional development efforts. That made for some long silences in the beginning. Carol and I, however, expected teachers to bring their questions and insights to fuel the conversations. At the third meeting, in November, I took some of the meeting time to talk about teacher reflection, inquiry, theory-building, and about teacher inquiry being central to good teaching. That explicit talk about expectations seemed to encourage discussion. At the end of each meeting, group members identified one or two tasks to do before the next meeting. The agenda for the following meeting was shaped by these "homework" tasks.

Carol and I also e-mailed summaries of each meeting to all the Bladerunners. They also built a website where the work of the group could be posted—notes, useful Internet links, handouts, etc. It was always accessible, and anyone could contribute.

Another transformative exchange was our journaling. Each participant received a blank book, and at the beginning of each session, everyone wrote about what they had seen students do and about their new questions and insights. This expectation to write offers a potentially powerful exchange.

As the discussions progressed, the group generated a list of descriptors of "Great Connections"—our targeted comprehension strategy. This list provided criteria for evaluating students' comprehension connections, and we shaped the list into rubrics for teacher observation and for students' self-evaluation. It is now February of our first year together, and each teacher is using and adapting the rubrics for use with various groups of students and for various kinds of reading. This provides a potential exchange, not only among the teachers, but among students as well. Connected with this is the use of "anchor charts"—or classroom charts that display these criteria—a potential transformative exchange with students.

By the fifth meeting, we began talking about how to share what we were learning with other teachers. Someone jokingly suggested that we should write a book, and we talked about developing presentations for local and state conferences. Soon, the opportunity to write this article came along.

Other, less structured, transformative exchanges happened daily. These teachers are colleagues in a fairly small school, and they see one another every day. They teach one another's children and shop at the same stores. This particular professional development project is just one more opportunity for conversation— a chance for focused conversation and collaborative inquiry.

It is the complex dynamics across all these exchanges that make self-organization possible.

What Are We Learning?

We are learning about how to teach comprehension and composition strategies, but we are also learning about how we can influence the interdependent conditions of self-organizing systems to sustain our collaborative inquiry. We are learning that self-organization will not continue if we don't feel like a "group." We are learning how important it is to have multiple ways to read, write, talk, and think about the significant differences across our work. We are also learning that this work applies to self-organization among teachers, among students, and within the thinking of individuals as they build their personal theories.

At every opportunity, Carol and I not only attempt to reinforce group identify but also to emphasize significant differences. We try to downplay irrelevant or distracting differences across the group. We try to focus and emphasize the differences that we judge will make a difference for the students' literacy. We have planned for multiple ways that teachers can teach and learn together. Some are regularly scheduled, with predictable structures, and some are spontaneous. Some are written, and some are face-to-face; some with immediate feedback and some with built-in wait time.

The conditions of self-organizing systems can help us explain and influence these dynamics. When participants are aware of these conditions, they can make informed decisions about how to help groups build shared identity; about how to focus on significant differences; and about how to set up potentially powerful transformative exchanges. When participants are aware of these conditions, they have a language to use as they negotiate goals, agendas, schedules and tasks. They have tools for problem-solving when things go wrong.

Because "questions of practice are not simple, predictable or standardized," those of us who work in schools must find ways to work together to build self-sustaining teaching/learning systems. Case studies like this suggest that it is possible. What we know about the conditions of self-organizing systems can help us learn to influence human system dynamics. What we are learning can help us sustain our individual and collaborative inquiries. And those inquiries can help us move beyond "bureaucratic solutions" to give our students the support they need.

Leslie Patterson, Ph.D.
After nine years of teaching English and speech in public schools, grades 7–12, Leslie joined the ranks of university-based teacher educators in 1987. Since then, she has taught Texas teachers and prospective teachers at three universities. She currently teaches in the College of Education at the University of North Texas. Her work as a teacher researcher and as a

facilitator of teacher research among K–12 teachers has yielded a number of collaborative publications. Her current research focuses on professional learning networks among teachers.

Carol Wickstrom, Ph.D.

Dr. Carol Wickstrom is currently on the Reading Program faculty at the University of North Texas. She teaches graduate and undergraduate courses in literacy assessment, language arts methods, and writing. She is Co-Director of the newly established North Star of Texas Writing Project—a National Writing Project site. Prior to teaching at the university level she taught first through sixth grade and special education for twenty years. Her current focus is to integrate theory and practice in collaborative research with teachers as they strive to make informed decisions in response to the needs of their students.

This article was written in collaboration with the reading and English faculty at Decatur Middle School, in Decatur, Texas. Dr. J. Kennedy, the superintendent of Decatur Independent School District, supports the on-going work of these teachers. The principal is Linda Whiddon, and the school improvement consultant is Pam Holland. The teachers who did the real work are Debbie Boatright, Jody Carter, Sonja Edwards, Randy Freeman, Mollie Furrh, Lisa Heiens, Julie Keith, and Elizabeth Luttmer.

ORGANIZATIONAL ADAPTATION

COMPLEXITY GIVES US THE CONCEPT "EQUIFINALITY," WHICH ALLOWS FOR MULTIPLE EQUIVALENT PATHS TO THE SAME OUTCOME. IN REAL LEADERSHIP SITUATIONS, THOUGH, NOT ALL PATHS ARE CREATED EQUAL. THE MULTIPLICITY OF PATHS MAY LEAD TO BLIND ALLEYS AND CLIFF EDGES. DENNIS CHEESEBROW'S LEADERSHIP FRAMEWORKS PROVIDE MAPS FOR GROUP CONVERSATION, DECISION MAKING, AND ACTION. THESE MAPS ARE DISTINCT ENOUGH TO SHAPE PROCESS, BUT NOT SO DEFINITIVE AS TO CONSTRAIN GENERATIVE SELF-ORGANIZING PROCESSES. BASED ON THE CDE MODEL FOR SELF-ORGANIZING IN HUMAN SYSTEMS AND YEARS OF PRACTICE AS AN EXPERT LEADER AND FACILITATOR, THE FRAMEWORKS FOCUS CONVERSATIONS AND HELP A GROUP MOVE TOWARD COORDINATED ACTION.

LEADING ORGANIZATIONS IN NEW WAYS

By Dennis Cheesebrow

Leaders in the 21st century organization are being confronted and challenged by a wide array of dynamic and changing expectations, temptations, opportunities, and illusions. The expectations of the past (a gradual path of increasing responsibilities and skills in supervisory management through executive management) have been reshaped by dramatic shifts in cultural, economic, and organizational aspects of organizations. The hierarchical leadership styles of yesterday have been complemented by the participative style of today and the learning organization style of the near future. In fact, many leaders in today's organizations realize and accept that they need to be adept in all four distinct forms of leadership: Hierarchical, Institutional, Participative, and Learning. An added key to success is the flexibility to shape one's style to the leadership needs of the moment.

In the Old Days	In the New Days
Organizations appeared to be controllable	Organizations appear as a series of interrelated, emerging and diminishing patterns
Control was achieved through tight connections	Control is achieved through loose connections
Machine metaphors shaped the image and language	Organic metaphors shape the image and language
Strategic planning and predictability	Strategic frameworks and adaptability
Linear, concrete sequential thinking	Nonlinear, patterned, and emergent thinking
Components and equilibrium thinking	Systems and human dynamics thinking
Leaders as heroes and larger than life	Leaders as enablers that live authentic lives

In the new days, leaders are being asked to challenge and change many of the cultural, institutional, and functional characteristics of leadership and to lead in a new way. A new tool set has emerged, and both theory and application tools are generating a new understanding of leadership and new leadership practices.

The field of human systems dynamics has been described as the application of the principles of chaos and complexity to human interaction, in both work and play. Several emerging application tools have been developed that make the theory usable and useful. Theory and practice have been merged over the past few years to transform the skills and approaches of leadership. In for-profit, non-profit, government, education organizations and religious institutions, this combination of theory and practice is being developed, shared, and applied. This new set of tools can be thought of as a collection of Leadership Frameworks for leadership thought and action.

The frameworks have emerged in concert with the CDE Model (Container, Difference, Exchange) of human systems dynamics created by Glenda Eoyang and presented in *Facilitating Organizational Change*. The CDE Model posits that three conditions are critical for the self-organization of human systems and effective work of change agents within those organizations:

1. The container must be clearly defined and continually clarified and redefined.

2. The system state is most influenced by the "differences that make a difference," the leverage points for change and transition that are most critical to be known and understood.

3. The transforming exchanges are vehicles through which a human system engages in transition, learning, and change.

Any organization or group includes "change agents" who can initiate change and/or be accountable for guiding and managing change. The leader who guides an organization is more effective if the role and power of the change agent is understood, valued, and practiced through processes and viewpoints that enable transforming exchanges in the organization.

Leadership Frameworks define and demonstrate multiple viewpoints and tools that support a leadership practice of seeing and defining the container, of identifying and leveraging the key differences and finally, the practical processes of engaging in transformational exchanges for the individual, the group, and the organization.

The common characteristics of "frameworks" are:

- *Frameworks are graphical images.* The images are simple and memorable. They mirror most people's reality and experience to form common language and symbols.

- *Frameworks are "content-less."* The graphics are a process map. The content and substance are provided by the current situations and environment. The "content-less" characteristic allows for broad application and flexibility in use.

- *Frameworks are dynamic and provide a sense of movement and action.* They reinforce the image of leadership as an on-going interaction with an organization, rather than a static imposition of power or allocation of resources.

- *Frameworks are flexible and adaptable.* The image can be translated across language and individual differences and be applied in a wide variety of situations and to a wide variety of challenges.

Leaders need practical and effective tools for "seeing" and assessing system-level change and growth in an organization as well as tools for action in the daily work of leadership. A Framework is a graphical image that depicts both process and viewpoint, or a frame of reference through which one can interpret the complex web of situations, environments, intentions, influences, and actions.

The table below illustrates how the Leadership Frameworks developed by TeamWorks International, Inc. are aligned with the CDE Model and how they play out in the behaviors and responsibilities of leadership.

CDE Model	Leadership Frameworks	Leadership Function
Container	Growth, Transition, and Change	See and map a system of change
	Whole System View	Systems assessment and strategies
	Organizational Change	Governance development, managing organizational transition, and change
Difference	Decision Making	Mapping of process, roles, authority
	Personal Growth and Change	Mapping of process of internal leadership growth and change
Exchange	Participation	Process of basic conversation, creative solutions, consensus and commitment to action and ownership
	Operating in the Now	Leadership stance choices

With the overview of the Frameworks and how they are exhibited in the function of leadership, it may be helpful to go more deeply into each of the Frameworks and see how each applies to real-world situations.

Growth, Transition, and Change Framework (GTC) allows for mapping, planning, and seeing patterns in the complex array of formal and informal change initiatives and influences in organizations.

How can I map out the organizational life of change so that "chaos and confusion" does not reign and so that an appreciation for the natural flow of change and continuous improvement can permeate and constructively influence this organization?"

GTC provides a single point view of the organizational "container," the key points for critical "exchange" and illuminates the different types of work needed for both integrating change and identifying the components of the system that need to be diminished and replaced. A school district mapped out over 80 existing change initiatives, organized the initiatives into "streams of changes" from the Shadow Zone to the Public Zone, and saw patterns and differences of success, failure and resistance. Strategies for managing change were developed and implemented. A large medical care provider mapped out the external and internal forces and groups that resisted and supported change initiatives. They developed clear staffing and leadership development strategies. A large insurance company in the midst of merger and reorganization identified key influences of change and developed a strategic framework for the internal IT group while business groups were developing merger strategies in parallel.

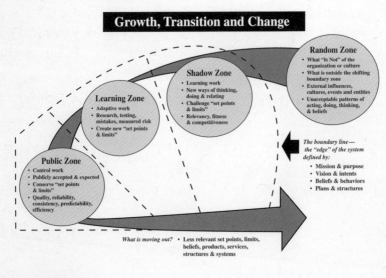

Growth, Transition and Change

Random Zone
- What "Is Not" of the organization or culture
- What is outside the shifting boundary zone
- External influences, cultures, events and entities
- Unacceptable patterns of acting, doing, thinking, & beliefs

Shadow Zone
- Learning work
- New ways of thinking, doing & relating
- Challenge "set points & limits"
- Relevancy, fitness & competitiveness

Learning Zone
- Adaptive work
- Research, testing, mistakes, measured risk
- Create new "set points & limits"

Public Zone
- Control work
- Publicly accepted & expected
- Conserve "set points & limits"
- Quality, reliability, consistency, predictability, efficiency

The boundary line — the "edge" of the system defined by:
- Mission & purpose
- Vision & intents
- Beliefs & behaviors
- Plans & structures

What is moving out? • Less relevant set points, limits, beliefs, products, services, structures & systems

Whole System View Framework (WSV) provides for quick and comprehensive situation, issue and opportunity assessment that leads to effective and focused strategies for allocation of resources.

How can I make sense out of opportunities and challenges that seem to defy conventional wisdom and practice? What is a quick, thorough, and consistent process of thinking and assessment?

WSV helps articulate the "container," the key "differences," and the critical interdependencies and relationships among the "differences."

An executive team of a large health care provider completed a comprehensive assessment of a public relations crisis in a short time. They developed sound systemic strategies for internal and external response. A project manager assessed true "differences" of a project team that were leading to internal conflict and project failure. A state government central agency assessed current reality in a creative and collaborative manner when faced with a substantial funding cutback. They began to identify successful strategies for re-structuring services, resources, and operating culture.

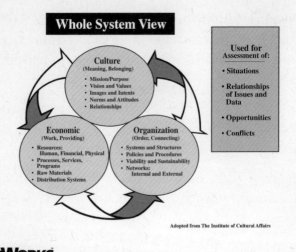

Organizational Change Framework (OC) enables leaders to fulfill their roles by establishing the critical components of the environment that allow for the creative and timely action of the organization.

What are some simple patterns of leadership that provide both accountability and creativity? How can a leader's actions be aligned with roles and responsibilities in a way that is less time consuming, stressful, and confusing?

When leaders establish the context, goals, and boundaries of unacceptable means, they establish clear accountability for the work of the organization while working within their own roles. Multiple governance boards have used this framework to understand their roles and relationships to management. They have come to see how policies and procedures mesh to form an environment in which creative and collaborative work can occur. A for-profit laboratory manager re-structured his work with a research team to improve time management and goal achievement while attending fewer meetings. Managers have been better able to fulfill their roles of setting context, outcomes, and boundaries and then allowing work teams and departments to create innovative and effective means of accomplishment.

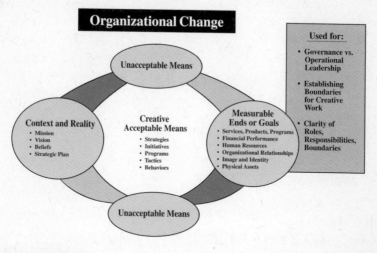

Organizational Change

Unacceptable Means

Context and Reality
- Mission
- Vision
- Beliefs
- Strategic Plan

Creative Acceptable Means
- Strategies
- Initiatives
- Programs
- Tactics
- Behaviors

Measurable Ends or Goals
- Services, Products, Programs
- Financial Performance
- Human Resources
- Organizational Relationships
- Image and Identity
- Physical Assets

Used for:
- Governance vs. Operational Leadership
- Establishing Boundaries for Creative Work
- Clarity of Roles, Responsibilities, Boundaries

Unacceptable Means

TEAMWORKS INTERNATIONAL, INC.

Decision Making Framework (DMF) helps identify roles, authority, expectations, and timing for the decision-making process. This leads to implementation and refinement of change.

How can I get my organization, and myself, unstuck from our cultural and political influences and patterns of working so that we accept authority, find solutions that satisfy, and escape endless studies or other delay tactics?

The process introduces the concept of choice making as a critical step in a decision-making process. This Framework provides a clear process to create focus and understanding of internal staff and external stakeholders regarding who gets to do what and when. Each participant understands why he or she can't make the decision alone.

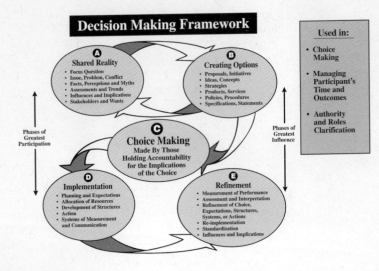

Participation Framework (PF) is a foundational process of dialogue and the development of shared meaning and problem solving in human systems. It is a flexible and scalable Framework that applies to conversations, planning, conflict resolution, conferences, retreats, and conciliation processes.

How can I release and engage the talent, intelligence, and good will of the organization? How can we break through patterns of inertia, resistance to change, and outright insubordination?

This Framework has transformed leaders' understanding of professional and personal relationships, and of the act of leadership in developing consensus and commitment. It provides a simple, scalable, and flexible process tool that can be used in the boardroom or the bathroom, in the hallway or the parking lot.

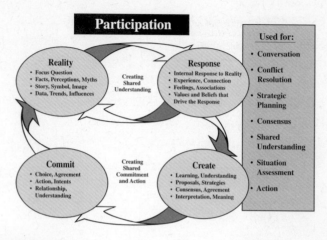

Personal Growth and Change Framework (PGC) is the personal parallel to the other frameworks. It takes advantage of the fact that organizational change occurs in concert with personal growth and change.

In the midst of all of this leadership stuff and my focus on guiding others, what about me? How can I reflect on my own journey of growth, transition, and change? How can I effectively develop the internal side of leadership while others experience my external journey?

The framework allows individuals and groups to map the process of personal change. It provides an assessment to identify barriers and limits to change. A school district used the framework to discover that an important curriculum change was unsuccessful because the success depended upon who had conducted the orientation and training. When leaders and their organizations understand what changes are not possible, they save professional development and intervention resources for other, more possible, changes. A senior executive consistently created high impact and negative events in key presentations and verbal exchanges with clients. When this framework was used in coaching setting the individual was able to identify learning and language limitations that could be addressed in a timely or effective manner. Alternative career choices enabled the this person to move into a well-matched position with more rewarding aspects for the individual and the organization.

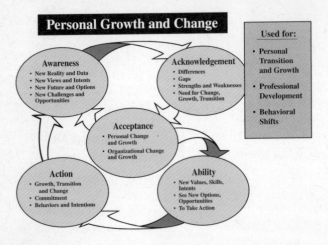

Operating in the Now Framework (OITN) provides a clear and challenging tool for individuals and groups to be intentional about how they "frame" the "exchanges" that affect the organization.

How might we operate without the confines of "we tried that" and "that might be risky"? How can we move into a reality where we deal with the issues, opportunities, and challenges at hand. How can my organization be engaged in the current reality while learning from the past and planning for the future?

OITN provides insight into the influence and limitations of operating in either the past or the future, and provides behavioral choices for operating in the present.

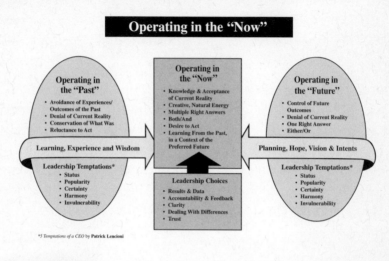

Dennis Cheesebrow

Dennis Cheesebrow serves as the Director of Services for the Human Systems Dynamics Institute, a non-profit organization whose mission is to facilitate the development of theory and practice in the field of human systems dynamics.

Dennis is also the principal coach and consultant of TeamWorks International, Inc., an organizational development and learning practice that guides individuals and groups through growth, transition and, change.

Clients most often find value in the creativity and inclusiveness of the processes, comfort and ease of his work with diverse groups, energy and humor in accomplishing the goals, and effective and efficient use of an organization's time and resources.

His client-referral practice spans many markets and applications in for-profit corporations and business, non-profit organizations and religious institutions, and education and government entities.

With a background and experience in product research and development, manufacturing and quality improvement, marketing, business management, project management and strategic planning, Dennis augments his mechanical engineering education with practical experience and learning to speak many of the organizational "languages" present in today's workplaces.

Dennis has also served as an adjunct professor with the School of Education and Murray Institute at the University of St. Thomas in Minneapolis, Minnesota and as a qualified trainer for the Technology of Participation courses through the Institute of Cultural Affairs.

EFFICIENT AND EQUITABLE DELIVERY OF HUMAN SERVICES HAS ALWAYS BEEN A CHALLENGE FOR EVERY LEVEL OF GOVERNMENT. INDIVIDUALS NEED HELP. SOME INDIVIDUALS LIVE AND WORK IN FAMILIES AND COMMUNITIES THAT MAY PROVIDE SUPPORT; OTHERS IN FAMILIES AND COMMUNITIES THAT MAY MAKE MATTERS WORSE. OVER TIME, BUREAUCRATIC SYSTEMS HAVE EMERGED THAT TRY TO DELIVER SERVICES WHEN AND WHERE THEY ARE NEEDED, BUT CURRENT CHANGES IN POLITICAL, CULTURAL, AND ECONOMIC CLIMATES DEMAND NEW AND MORE ADAPTIVE STRUCTURES AND FUNCTIONS. IN THIS ARTICLE, YELLOWTHUNDER AND WARD APPLY THE CDE MODEL TO EXPLORE OPTIONS FOR MORE INTEGRATED AND EFFECTIVE DELIVERY OF SERVICES.

Designing and Implementing Organizational Change in a Complex Adaptive System

By Lois Yellowthunder, Ph.D. and Vic Ward

Introduction

Metropolis (a pseudonym for a large, urban county in the upper Midwest) Neighborhood Services (MNS), is a neighborhood based multidisciplinary team of health and human services workers, and part of Metropolis County's broader effort to integrate services to promote better results for children and families. We will use the creation and implementation of MNS to illustrate how Glenda Eoyang's CDE Model applied to human systems dynamics within a complexity framework can be used for analyzing and evaluating a change process as well as setting the conditions for change.

Recent research in organizational management, behavior, and psychology indicate that many human systems behave as complex adaptive systems (CAS). "A complex adaptive system behaves/evolves according to three key principles:

1. Order is emergent as opposed to hierarchical

2. The system's history is irreversible

3. The system's future is often unpredictable.

The basic building blocks of the CAS are agents." Prediction and controlled performance toward a goal cannot be expected from a complex adaptive system. Unlike other types of systems, it is neither Organized nor Unorganized (chaotic), but rather Self-organizing. The number of agents (in this case, people and governmental agencies) drives constant change in this situation. Interacting agents form patterns. There are also interdependencies between the agents and their environments. These complex interactions generate a system that is roiling with change.

The common perception, however, is that these human systems are either organized or, at times, chaotic. The former is highly desired the latter is seen as threatening. Analytic frameworks, change strategies or methodologies and system interventions all reflect these perceptions as implicit assumptions. Accordingly, change is viewed as a linear process that can be directed toward achieving pre-determined goals and outcomes — thus eliminating uncertainty and potential chaos. The process, it is believed, can then be evaluated by the quality and degree to which these pre-determined goals and outcomes are met. MNS was developed within such a process that set general goals and expectations and assumed these would be achieved through linear planning and development. As previously indicated, human systems do not move inexorably toward a project's end point. They may not come to rest even when the end of a project is reached. A manager may be able to assign an arbitrary beginning and end date of an intervention, but the system itself recognizes no such boundaries in time. For this reason, the whole concept of projected and predictable outcomes is an artificial construct in a CAS. A manager may be able to frame expectations, but the self-organizing nature of the system may result in completely different outcomes than those expected. This environment requires new tools. By viewing the planning, development, and implementation of MNS through a complexity lens and applying dynamic tools we are able to work with a decision model that we believe more closely mirrors the real world and sets the conditions for change.

Glenda Eoyang has designed a model, which identifies three conditions for self-organization of human systems. These conditions are: Containers (C), Differences that make a difference (D) and Exchanges (E). The particular configuration of Containers, Differences and Exchanges forms a pattern. In this essay we show how decision-makers could have applied this model to the development of Metropolis Neighborhood Services by asking five questions. The questions are:

1. What is the existing pattern?

2. What CDE conditions led to the existing pattern?

3. What pattern do the decision-makers want?

4. What actions could move the system to self-organize toward the desired pattern?

5. What are the recommended actions?

We will demonstrate that the CDE Model developed by Glenda Eoyang, together with the five questions listed above, can be used to inform the design, implementation, and evaluation of the change process for MNS. We also believe it has great utility for change processes in complex adaptive systems in general.

Background of Metropolis Neighborhood Services

In 1997 the Coordinated Services Group (CSG) was formed. CSG included members from the following Metropolis County Departments: Adult Services, Children and Family Services, Coordinated Corrections, Coordinated Health, Economic Assistance, Policy Center, Metropolis County Medical Center, Primary Care, Training and Employment Assistance, and Veterans Services. The number of departments as well as their numerous interdependencies around common clients indicates the complexity of the environment from which MNS emerged. While having many common interests, these Departments, like agents of the complex adaptive systems' model, had surprisingly diverse and sometimes contradictory objectives for the project.

MNS was characterized from the first by both innovation and current structure/practices. A multidisciplinary team in a neighborhood office with a dynamic and creative program coordinator represented innovation and change, while the underlying administrative structure replicating the larger county organization represented the status quo.

Six CSG departments contributed staff to MNS. Throughout its development and implementation, each department maintained control over its employees. Thus department affiliation continued to be a significant difference. Another significant difference—debated and challenged at MNS—was professional versus non-professional status. Traditional organizational structure, supervision, hierarchy, compensation, patterns of practice, and funding emerge from these differences. At MNS, the project coordinator devoted a significant amount of time and resources to managing these traditional differences while at the same time trying to create an innovative cross-functional environment.

The Eoyang CDE Model

At Metropolis Neighborhood Services the County staff, community service providers, and the clients became part of a self-organized solution to the problem. The Coordinated Services Group, CSG, set the course, but the project coordinator and the multidisciplinary team members made MNS a successful enterprise. Since MNS's inception in 1998, clients living and working in the neighborhood served by MNS experienced a different relationship with Metropolis County.

The whole person became the central focus of workers' activities rather than parsing out particular individual needs to particular services. Integrated services meant that the client had access to the appropriate combination of services. The neighborhood location and a staff more familiar with neighborhood resources meant that clients could use Metropolis County and neighborhood services in a more convenient, coordinated fashion. This was a significant change from the past, or, in CDE terms, a difference that makes a difference. MNS staff members self-organized around the new concepts of focusing on the whole person in their living environment, integrated services in a neighborhood location, and a multidisciplinary team.

As noted above, the CDE Model posits three conditions that shape self-organization. They are:

- Containers (C) which provides boundaries for the system. Boundaries are of two types: external boundaries such as physical spaces and an attractor ("a pattern that emerges through time in a chaotic system") such as a visionary leader or motivating goal.

- Differences (D), these are distinctions within a system that establishes a potentially generative tension and can create new containers. They represent the potential for change. Organizational examples include power, resources, language, and mission.

- Exchanges (E) which is a transfer of information, resources or energy between agents that results in changes within the agents and/or changes in system-wide patterns. Examples include financial transactions, surveys, and conversations. These three components are defined as the "conditions for self-organizing in human systems."

The table below, The CDE Model, shows how decisions can be made. The shaded areas in the table show how Metropolis County services looked before the CSG decided to develop MNS.

CDE Model

	Organized	Self-organizing	Unorganized
Container	Few, Small	Many, Entangled	Large, Many
Difference	Few	Many, Some significant	Innumerable
Exchange	Tight, Clear	Loose, Ambiguous	Arbitrary, Meaningless

If a decision-maker or a decision-making team wanted to make a change in a complex adaptive system, such as Metropolis County's delivery of services, they have a choice of many actions — any one of which could potentially move the current pattern from either Organized or Unorganized to Self-organizing. Decision-makers could decide to make a container change. Some of the types of action that will affect containers are assigning smaller teams, offering services from one place, offering fewer services, or dealing with both the client and family as a unit of service.

Another possible set of actions would be to reduce the number of differences thus moving the expected pattern from the Unorganized to Self-organizing columns. Some possible way to accomplish this would be through improved access to decision support information, integrated client services or greater familiarity with the community. Finally, decision-makers might act to change the exchange conditions of the pattern. They might talk with people face to face, build relationships with family and residents, or encourage engagement among staff. In a general sense, these decisions answer the question, what actions will shift the conditions and therefore stimulate movement toward a new and more effective pattern?

To demonstrate how the CDE Model can be used to inform the design, implementation, and evaluation of change processes in complex adaptive systems, we will apply the five questions posed at the beginning of this essay to MNS. We will illustrate their use for three phases of the process: design, implementation, and evaluation. We will use tables to show the components of a pattern in a simplified manner.

Design Phase (CSG and other decision makers)

1. What is the existing pattern?

Identify the pattern (current self-organized state that constitutes the whole system: multiple agents, levels, building structures of different kinds) that currently exists, e.g., too much money spent, geographic concentration of clients, competition among departments, families lost in the process. During this phase of the process the decision-makers determine if the part of the environment that needs to change is Organized, Self-organizing, or Unorganized. The Pattern Diagnostic Tool shown in the table below helps decision-makers identify the conditions of the existing pattern.

Pattern Diagnosis Tool for the Existing Pattern of Service Delivery before MNS

Conditions for Self-organization	Organized	Self-organizing	Unorganized
Container	*Small and few*	*Many and entangled*	*Large and many*
Difference	*Few*	Many, some Significant	*Innumerable*
Exchange	*Tight*	*Loose*	*Arbitrary*
	Clear	Ambiguous (fax, copier, computer)	Meaningless
Emergent behavior	*Predictable patterns*	*Emergent patterns*	*No patterns*
	Rigid Structure Linear cause and effect Tight coupling	Emergent structure Nonlinear cause and effect Loose coupling	Random No cause and effect Uncoupling

2. What CDE conditions led to the existing pattern?

What is keeping the current system/pattern in place? A lot of resources are going into maintaining the status quo, therefore, what processes, people or structures maintain the status quo? The table below shows another way to look at the situation is to look at the layers/levels of organization; costs and outcomes.

Pattern of Service Delivery Examined by CSG

Existing Container	Existing Differences	Existing Exchanges
Human Service Delivery System	Fed, State, County	Legislation, regulation and funds
Metropolis County	Departments Lines of Business	County-wide strategic planning County Board conversations County Administrator
CSG Departments	HSG and others Individual departments Health and others	Budgeting Resource allocation Planning Procedures Projects
CSG Directors' Group	Departments Personal power bases Time in job Experience on the line Connections to Commissioners	Weekly meetings Email/minutes/reports
Individual Director	Performance expectations Relationships with employees Understanding of process Identity with turf	Conversations with persons within and outside department
Department	Eligibility rules Required procedures Funding streams Professional cultures (e.g., financial workers/social workers) Number of employees Physical location of employees Growing or shrinking resources	Workgroup meetings Formal and informal communications from Director Roles of middle managers
CSG Change Process	Perceptions of common issues Procedures with common clients Experiences with integration Current reality and overarching objectives Old skills and new skills Expectations for performance	Action Conference Shared outcomes initiatives On-line conferencing Thinking and Doing Sessions Training Outcomes, indicators, measures

3. What pattern did CSG want?

Examples of emergent behavior that CSG sought included integrated services, neighborhood-based service, and services delivered by a multidisciplinary team. To achieve those ends, the new pattern they envisioned shifted the service delivery from "Metropolis County" to one labeled "Neighborhood Office," illustrated by the table below.

New Pattern

Container	Difference	Exchange
Metropolis County	Single case file	Encourage engagement among staff
Neighborhood Office	Small team Single place Integrated Services Client and family as a unit	Build relationship with families and residents Teach and learn in interactions

4. What actions could move the system to self-organize towards the desired pattern?

A number of actions could move the system to self-organize toward the desired pattern. They include establishing a neighborhood based center which changes the container, setting up a multidisciplinary team made up of employees from various provider departments which changes differences, and changing the service delivery location to a neighborhood which changes the exchanges.

5. What are the recommended actions?

The recommendations from the Design Phase were to move from the existing system toward a self-organizing system with a number of dimensions:

- Staff was to remain administratively attached to their original departments (this replicates the larger system).

- Establish a multidisciplinary team and locate it in a neighborhood where the clients lived.

- Maintain a strong relationship with community service providers (by working more collaboratively together and doing better coordinating with common clients).

- Offer more than one service to clients if more services are needed.

- Include families and neighbors of clients when working with clients, if needed.

- Residents, families and neighbors of clients are to be provided with consultation and information and referral services.

In the next phase of the MNS project, the CDE Model was applied to the work done at the Metropolis Neighborhood Services as a neighborhood service delivery organization. In reality, CSG did carry out a number of actions that fit into the CDE Model. These included:

- Creating smaller containers including team, neighborhood office, geographic area served

- Focusing on significant differences such as how clients are selected and served, who is served (families, neighbors of clients)

- Establishing transforming exchanges across disciplines, programs and departments.

Implementation Phase (Metropolis Neighborhood Services staff and neighborhood service providers)

1. What is the existing pattern?
This is the same table as the one in the Design Phase, step 2, "Pattern of Service Delivery Examined by CSG."

2. What CDE led to the current situation?
What is keeping the current pattern in place? The pattern of service delivery that existed before MNS was characterized by a central location in downtown

Metropolis for most clients to go to. (There were some regional offices for specialized services.) In a number of cases, service coordination was problematic. Work rules were less flexible.

3. What pattern do the decision-makers want?

The recommendations were made by CSG in the Design Phase. The table below shows the desired pattern.

CSG Desired Pattern

Desired Container	Desired Difference	Desired Exchange
Neighborhood	Neighbors and family members can meet with staff, I&R	Information sharing Staff participation in community events
County	Integrated Disciplines/ departments/programs working together (multi-disciplinary team)	Electronic common case management system Case consultation
Non-profit	Proximity	Collaboration
Other jurisdictions	Proximity	Collaboration
Neighborhood		Staff becomes familiar with client surroundings

4. What actions could move the system to self-organize toward the desired pattern?

MNS staff could familiarize themselves with community services and other resources available to the clients. They could introduce community providers to Metropolis County programs. They could restrict MNS's client base to a specific neighborhood. They could establish one point of contact between the client and MNS, preferably the first staff person the client meets with during the initial contact.

To change the existing pattern of service delivery, MNS staff could change eligibility requirements, integrate services (that is, change the definition of a case), change the relationship with neighborhood services, use multidisciplinary case consultation to decide the need for services, and let the original staff contact manage the client throughout his or her involvement with the service delivery system.

5. What are the recommended actions?

In terms of the CDE Model, MNS staff and management are to implement a number of changes:

- Set the container conditions by conducting client contact and meeting in a new neighborhood storefront and revising the definition of a case to family and/or service mix.

- Set the difference conditions of the new service delivery pattern by establishing the policy that eligibility doesn't always determine the service that is received and that professional/non-professional status doesn't always determine who works with people.

- Set the exchange conditions by changing the way case consultation is conducted and changing to a common electronic case management system.

Metropolis Neighborhood Services organized around the innovative recommendations set by CSG. The project coordinator, the staff at MNS, and local service providers set the conditions to make Metropolis Neighborhood Services successful by offering integrated, client-focused services to neighborhood clients.

Evaluation Phase—Applying the Lessons Learned from MNS (CSG and staff from other organizations that will operate under new guidelines)

1. What is the desired pattern?

See the table, CSG Desired Pattern, from the Implementation Phase, question 3, above.

2. How well does the MNS pattern fit with the desired pattern?

The CSG would need to answer the following question: Did MNS accomplish the desired pattern conditions described in Implementation Phase, step 3? If MNS succeeded then proceed with the following steps. If more work is needed then a new iteration of the process with the five questions could be initiated.

3. What pattern does CSG want based on lessons from MNS?

In the following table CSG would fill in the conditions it decided were successful at MNS.

Table 6 Desired Pattern

Container	Difference	Exchange

4. What actions could move the system to self-organize toward the desired pattern?

To decide what CDE conditions need changing, Metropolis County could develop a community-based mediation process to implement the lessons in other places with a new set of County staff, community service providers, and clients. This process would change the transforming exchanges as well as the significant differences. Mediation (using the Harvard Negotiation Model) is a decision-making process that implicitly uses the CDE Model defined as the conditions for self-organizing in human systems. It is a self-organizing process that explicitly states that there is more than one right answer and there are multiple solutions, which could be mutually beneficial. The process is predictive in the sense that, at its conclusion, the participants will either reach agreement on what action to take or acknowledge that no agreement can be reached.

5. What are the recommended actions?
The proposed actions would come from the mediation process described above.

Another phase could be started here or the project could be left alone. An iterative process can be used for as many phases as the decision-makers want. The beauty of the CDE Model is that change is acknowledged and embraced.

Conclusion

In this article we have:

- Illustrated the development of Metropolis Neighborhood Services—a complex adaptive system—using the CDE Model

- Shown how this model describes the dynamics of MNS

- Suggested possible iterations

- Described the current situation as a pattern

- Generated new patterns to guide decision making

- Shown how to recognize when the real world situation has developed in the direction desired, or is moving toward another pattern

The CDE process applied to a real-world set of patterns provides the tools for analyzing the current pattern as well as the one that develops after suggested actions are implemented and the system starts to self-organize into a new pattern.

Lois Yellowthunder, Ph.D.

Lois Yellowthunder works as a health and human services planner and organization development consultant for Hennepin County (Minneapolis), Minnesota. Her original career goal was to be a Curator of Anthropology for a natural history museum. She worked for the Los Angeles Museum of Natural History, San Diego Museum of Man, the Field Museum of Natural History in Chicago and the Science Museum of Minnesota. County government is her second career. In addition to Hennepin County, she worked in five other metropolitan counties in Minnesota and California. Communities, neighborhoods, children, and families are a major focus of her work. Lois received her Ph.D. in Anthropology from the University of Minnesota, her M.A. in Anthropology from the University of Chicago and her B.A. in Anthropology from the University of California at Los Angeles. She is currently Adjunct Faculty in the Department of Family Social Science at the University of Minnesota.

Victor W. Ward

Vic Ward has worked with organizations of all types: for-profit, non-profit, educational, as well as governmental agencies. He has written a book on strategic planning and complex adaptive systems and helped to edit *Facilitating Organizational Change* by Glenda Eoyang and Ed Olson. He has also been a webmaster and helped organizations to research, develop, and maintain a presence on the world wide web.

Vic's teaching experience includes St. Mary's University, Management M.B.A. Program and he is currently a faculty member of Metropolitan State University, Department of Management, where he teaches in both the undergraduate and MBA programs. Prior to 1998, he worked in city planning and research in Texas, as Senior Planner and previously, as Manager of Economic Studies for the City of Dallas.

Vic holds a Master of Liberal Studies degree from St. Johns College, Santa Fe and BS degrees in Physics and Mathematics from Texas Tech University.

COMMUNITY ADAPTATION

ECONOMIC, AESTHETIC, ECOLOGICAL, AND CULTURAL
AGENDAS MEET HEAD-ON AS STAKEHOLDERS TRY TO
SHAPE PUBLIC POLICY AND PRACTICE AROUND THE
USE OF LAND AND WATER RESOURCES IN THE GRENADINE ISLANDS.
THIS TEAM'S STORY EXPLORES THE SELF-ORGANIZING NATURE OF
THE SYSTEM AND INVESTIGATES HOW THE CDE MODEL MIGHT
ILLUMINATE A PATH TOWARD SHARED PLANNING AND ACTION.

Coastal resources and livelihoods in the Grenadine Islands

By Sharon Almerigi, Robin Mahon, Patrick McConney, Cecil Ryan, Bryan Whyte

The Grenadine Islands, which lie on the Grenadine Bank and extend some 120 km between Grenada and St. Vincent, support the most extensive coral reefs and related habitats in the south-eastern Caribbean. The international boundary between Grenada and St. Vincent and the Grenadines lies about midway down the bank, which means they are shared by both countries. The largest islands have towns and communities. Others are resort islands. Most are visited by yachters and fishers. Tourism and fishing are the major sources of employment in the area.

Tourism development is proceeding apace, while fishery resources appear to be fully or over-exploited. Governments of both countries perceive their Grenadine Islands as having high potential for tourism and associated development. They also recognise the vulnerability of the marine and terrestrial ecosystems of the area to environmental degradation and that sustainable development depends on conservation of the resources. There, the emerging view is that the entire area should be a trans-boundary World Heritage Site. The Tobago Cays Marine Park has been established and other MPAs are planned, but a broader approach is needed. Achieving sustainable livelihoods from marine and coastal resources will need organizational change at many levels.

There is a complex interplay of local and international private interests, local, national, and international non-governmental organizations (NGOs) as well as tensions between main island government and local inhabitants. Therefore, conventionally planned change is difficult to implement. The model of organizational change that is most likely to be applicable is one based on the science of complex adaptive systems and chaos theory. Intervention should employ "containers,' 'significant differences,' and 'transforming exchanges' to increase the capacity for self-organization among stakeholders. Understanding of other chaos elements such as boundaries, butterfly effects, coupling, and attractors can also be used to encourage self-organization.

Development Potential and Problems

The entire Grenadines area is noted for its beautiful scenery, spectacular beaches, and diverse marine habitats that include coral reefs, mangroves, and seabird colonies. Tourism is a major source of employment and tourism development is proceeding. Private sector activities include: resorts, hotels, guest houses, restaurants, SCUBA dive operators, day and longer-term cruise operators, crafts, and shops. There are also under-utilised land-based opportunities for earnings through cultural and heritage developments that would diversify the tourism sector.

Fishing is the other major source of employment in the area and has long been a source of exports to neighboring islands.

Unplanned development and unregulated use of terrestrial and marine habitats and resources have already led to significant degradation in many areas. There are problems with:

- Over-fishing

- Near shore habitat destruction and degradation

- Terrestrial de-vegetation and overgrazing

- Sedimentation

- Solid waste disposal from land and boat sources

- Sewage disposal from land and boat sources

- Recreational abuse of coral reefs

There is no integrated framework within which to pursue development and conservation. Local governmental and non-governmental organizations lack the capacity to develop the framework or to participate fully in its development.

Biodiversity and Marine Resource Conservation

Marine resource and biodiversity conservation are fundamental to sustainable livelihoods in the Grenadines. These are in turn affected by the land use practices on the islands. Thus, it is necessary to consider both terrestrial and marine resource use practices in planning for biodiversity conservation.

The Government of SVG (GoSVG) has established the Tobago Cays Marine Park (TCMP) as both a major attraction and a means of conserving marine biodiversity. The TCMP is the focus of marine aquatic recreation (diving, day sailing, yachting) for the entire area. Private yachts visit the park and the area in general mainly from throughout the eastern Caribbean but also from beyond.

The TCMP was declared a regulated area in 1987 under the Fisheries Act, then supported by a Marine Parks Act in 1997, and regulations in 1998. There is a Board of Directors, a Park Manager and a Management Plan. However, there has been little progress with implementing the Plan and enforcing the regulations. The extent of involvement of local NGOs in the park and the capacity of the board and management unit are of concern for the success of the TCMP. Other Marine Protected Areas (MPAs) are being considered in other parts of the SVG Grenadines.

Several MPAs have also been identified as desirable for the Grenada Grenadines. These are proposed in an Integrated Physical Development and Environmental Management Plan for Carriacou and Petit Martinique prepared in 1998. Implementation of this plan has been hindered by lack of stakeholder buy-in and participation, and the capacity of NGOs to take part. One NGO, The Carriacou Environmental Committee, has taken the lead in establishing one of the MPAs off Hillsborough, Carriacou. Support through linkages with other MPAs, organizational capacity building, and access to technical information on MPAs would greatly facilitate its progress with the MPA.

Summary of the Situation

Inhabitants of the Grenadine Islands area are highly dependent on the marine environment for sustainable livelihoods. The area has the potential to sustain these livelihoods while contributing to the national economies and to regional and global biodiversity conservation. These potentials are presently being eroded by unplanned and uncoordinated development and continuing negative impacts of the resource users, both extractive and non-extractive. There is a need to reorient the stakeholders in the Grenadines towards sustainable use of the marine resources. Land-use issues have bearing on this too, and a holistic approach is needed. This reorientation will involve full engagement of the stakeholders in the process, including strengthening their capacity to take part in planning and decision-making processes, as well as in the implementation of the plans.

The Project

A project to facilitate change is being developed. The goal of the project is: The integrated sustainable development of the Grenadine Islands area for the social and economic well being of the people who live there, as a contributor to the national economies, and to conserve their biodiversity.

The primary purpose of this project is: To develop a participatory integrated sustainable development planning framework for the area and to implement those components of the plan that are directly associated with uses of the marine resources and environment.

A secondary purpose is: To develop a model for participatory integrated sustainable development in small island systems that can be adapted and applied elsewhere.

The goal and purpose are entirely consistent with, and guided by, several of the "Principles of environmental sustainability in the OECS" (OECS, 2001).

The Project Approach

The project is conceived for implementation in two phases:

Phase 1—Stakeholder assessment and participatory project development—will involve stakeholder assessment and mobilisation, including an appraisal of government and NGO capacity for participation. A participatory strategic planning process will be used to develop an integrated framework, and to generate the information required to prepare the proposal for the 5-year program to be implemented in Phase 2.

The outputs from Phase 1 will be:

- Increased stakeholder awareness and commitment for involvement

- Information on the relative interests and capacities of stakeholders

- Strategic and action plans

- Identification of the stakeholder alliances needed to effect continuous change towards sustainable development in the Grenadines

- Proposal for funding of the of the 5-year core project

- Related activities identified for subsequent proposal development

Phase 2—Implementation of the main elements of the 5-year core program—is expected to include a substantial institutional capacity building component for local NGOs and government departments. It will focus on the establishment of management and co-management systems required for sustainable resource use and management. There may be some elements of infrastructure development. It will also include the preparation of proposals for related elements that exceed the budget and immediate scope of the core project.

The Desired Impact of the Project

This integrated project is expected to have broad positive impacts on the conservation of marine resources and biodiversity in the Grenadines and on the sustainability of the livelihoods of the people who depend on those resources. It is expected to achieve this by:

- Strengthening the capacity of NGOs, government, and the private sector to work together to develop and implement projects

- Demonstrating the benefits of co-management arrangements where NGOs can become partners in the management of resources, such as fisheries and MPAs

- Increasing, throughout the Grenadines, an awareness of their dependency of marine resources, the vulnerability of the marine environment, and commitment to conservation and sustainable use

- Enhancing the environment for sustainable economic opportunities and development of both human and physical capital

- Providing multi-faceted linkages between individual, community, national, and trans-boundary developmental goals and the means of achieving their specific objectives

- Improving understanding by 'main island' government partners in St. Vincent and Grenada of the issues and special needs in the Grenadines

- Promoting the Grenadines nationally, regionally, and globally as a well-managed area of special scenic beauty and biodiversity

Change in Self-organizing Systems

Increasingly, the field of organization development is being influenced by breakthroughs in physics, biology, chemistry, and chaos theory which span several disciplines. A turning point was when Ilya Prigogene won the Nobel Prize in 1977 for demonstrating how certain chemical systems (dissipative structures) will regenerate to higher levels of self-organization in response to environmental demands.

Self-organization in human systems is explored by Olson and Eoyang (2001) in *Facilitating Organizational Change*. In *Coping with Chaos,* Eoyang (1997) makes the point that the17th century Newtonian world view no longer applies to today's fast-paced organizational dynamics. From the old view, managers tended to separate organizations into hierarchical parts, rely on exerting force for change, and to plan for a world that was expected to be predictable.

Through the new sciences a different world view is emerging—one that focuses on patterns and connections, and one that regards the whole of things and the importance of relationships (Wheatley, 1992). When this is applied to human organizations, change can be seen as a spontaneous, evolving, iterative process in which patterns emerge and influence behavior which then generate new patterns which influence further change.

Olson and Eoyang (2001) note that self-organization represents the tendency of a system to generate new structures and patterns based on its own internal dynamics. Pattern, in this context, refers to any coherent structure that emerges from a self-organizing process. In this mode, organization change patterns are not imposed from above or outside but emerge from the interactions of the agents of the system.

Because of human pressures and practices in the Grenadine Islands there has been some concern about whether patterns of sustainable development are emerging fast enough to offset environmental degradation. The agents of the system in the Grenadine Islands are its stakeholders: Government, private sector, and civil society (individuals and NGOs).

Left alone, organizations and groups will self-organize, but there is no guarantee that, in this case, those changes will be desirable; i.e. towards sustainable development in the context of this initiative. However, with an understanding of systems dynamics a change agent, who is internal or external to the system, may consciously influence the direction in which the system self-organizes.

Conventional change measures based on the Newtonian view are leader-driven, or top-down. However these measures often fail when they meet resistance from other participants in the system. In a self-organizing system the leader plays an important role, but long-lasting, meaningful change depends on the work of many individuals at different levels of the system.

Change agents who want to influence a system toward new and innovative patterns can formulate their inputs with reference to three system characteristics that are critical determinants of self-organization: **'container,' 'significant difference,' and 'transforming exchanges'** (Eoyang, 2001).

The concept of the **'container'** refers to the limits that define the self-organizing system or its sub-systems. A 'container' may be physical, as in a geographical area, organizational as in an NGO, or conceptual as in an identity, a shared vision, or an operating procedure. A system may be comprised of several containers which may overlap, and awareness of these is crucial to influencing change.

'Significant differences' are the differences that occur normally in systems, through heterogeneity or diversity. These 'significant differences' may relate to power, levels of expertise, gender, race, educational background, and so forth. The nature of these 'significant differences,' as well as the level to which they are appreciated, may greatly influence the emergence of beneficial patterns and structures.

'**Transforming exchanges**' consist of the active connections between participants in a system. These exchanges may include information, money, energy, or other resources that flow from person to person resulting in each of them being transformed in some way. Examples of transforming exchanges include meetings, emails, financial transactions, phone calls, etc. Feedback loops, or bidirectional exchanges, are particularly high impact transforming exchanges.

The conditions that are most favourable for self-organization are high diversity and active feedback. The Grenadines appears to be in a state of moderately high diversity and low feedback.

The table below illustrates organizational outcomes resulting from various combinations of organizational diversity and feedback (adapted from Eoyang 1997).

	High diversity	**Low diversity**
Active feedback loops	Self-organization	Reinforcement and revitalisation
No feedback loops	Unresolved conflict	Organizational rest

The Approach

The proposed approach to 'Sustainable Integrated Development and Biodiversity Conservation in the Grenadine Islands' will seek to encourage sustainable development by influencing the above three conditions for Grenadines stakeholders or system agents. Many of those stakeholders have been working toward sustainable development in isolation from each other. In particular, the larger system which spans the two countries to which the Grenadines belong is a recognisable, but poorly defined container.

To address the diffuse nature of the efforts thus far, this project will attempt to define or enhance 'containers' within which the system agents can be brought together. Containers may include the project framework itself, subprojects, meetings and various interest groups. Appreciation of the value of 'significant differences' will be enhanced by bringing together a number of people with different perspectives, experiences, and levels of expertise. 'Transforming exchanges' will be facilitated by an emphasis on participatory planning processes (generation of ideas and consensus building), and on communication networks.

Other aspects of chaos and complexity science can be applied when trying to facilitate change toward sustainable development. Facilitators of change towards sustainability through self-organization in complex systems such as the Grenadines Islands can benefit from an understanding of chaos and complexity science as applied to organizations.

Acknowledgements

We would like to thank The Lighthouse Foundation, Hamburg, Germany for supporting this work. We would also like to thank the participants from the government agencies of both countries, the many private individuals, and the numerous NGOs (too many to list) throughout the Grenadine Islands for their contribution to this work.

Sharon Almerigi

Sharon Almerigi is Principal Associate of People Dynamics Associates, Barbados and works as a facilitator and trainer for the private and public sectors as well as NGOs. She studied political science (Grand Valley State College, Michigan) and filmmaking (San Francisco Art Institute) and worked in film and radio, and journalism in California, Florida, and Grenada. Her current focus is in capacity building which includes leadership and conflict resolution training. She is a Certified Professional Facilitator through the International Association of Facilitators, a Qualified Trainer of Technology of Participation facilitation methods and co-founder of the Caribbean Facilitators Network.

Robin Mahon

Robin Mahon works at the Centre for Resource Management and Environmental Studies at the University of the West Indies in Barbados. He pursued his graduate studies in The University of Guelph in Canada and worked there with Fisheries and Oceans Canada for several years, returning to the Caribbean in 1986. He has worked extensively in fisheries and coastal management with FAO, CARICOM and as an independent consultant. Most recently he has been engaged in participatory co-management of coastal resources and in governance of the Caribbean Large Marine Ecosystem.

Patrick McConney

Patrick McConney works with the University of the West Indies and environmental non-governmental organizations in the Caribbean on coastal and marine matters, particularly from the perspectives of collaborative management and participatory approaches to decision-making. He was previously the head of the fisheries management authority in Barbados and holds an interdisciplinary doctorate in resource management from the University of British Columbia in Canada.

Brian Whyte

Born in Sauters, Grenada, Brian Whyte has a passion for the environment. He is a graduate of McDonald College, McGill University, Canada where he excelled in both academics and athletics. After moving to Carriacou (Grenada's sister island) in 1990, he co-founded the Carriacou Environmental Committee Inc. (CEC). Brian has been instrumental in CEC's drive to establish marine parks in Carriacou to preserve and protect the marine environment. He is committed to community and people empowerment as articulated by his membership on executive boards of the Carriacou Historical Society, the Carriacou Marketing Committee, the Carriacou Maroon Festival, and the Carriacou United Cricket Board.

DIFFERENCES OF PERSPECTIVE ARE THE FUEL FOR LEARNING, AND IN THIS CHAPTER FOUAD MIMOUNI PROVIDES SUFFICIENT FUEL FOR A BONFIRE. IN THIS THOUGHTFUL, WELL RESEARCHED AND REASONED PIECE, FOUAD EXPLORES THE SIMILARITIES AND DIFFERENCES BETWEEN AN ISLAMIC AND WESTERN VIEW OF COMPLEX ADAPTIVE AND SELF-ORGANIZING SYSTEMS. HIS ANALYSIS AND ARTICULATE DESCRIPTIONS REFLECT THE DYNAMICS OF HUMAN SYSTEMS ON A VARIETY OF LEVELS, FROM PHILOSOPHY AND METAPHYSICS, TO THEOLOGY, TO NATURAL SCIENCES, TO ETHICS AND AESTHETICS. THE DISTINCTIONS HE MAKES HELP CLARIFY THE LANDSCAPE OF COMPLEXITY AND MOVE OUR CONVERSATION ABOUT HUMAN SYSTEMS DYNAMICS FORWARD IN A VARIETY OF WAYS.

PURPOSEFUL SELF-ORGANIZATION AND MEANINGFUL EMERGENCE: A VOICE FROM ISLAM

By Fouad Mimouni

I am *(being) (re)* created, therefore I am.

Introduction

This article shares my reflections on the potential implications of the Islamic worldview on our understanding of human systems dynamics. After introducing two fundamental Islamic concepts relevant to the topic, namely *Tawhid* or the Unity of the Creator and causality, I will explore their implications on two other major concepts: intentionality and purposefulness. Then I will show how these four concepts help us understand human systems as complex adaptive systems in the light of the worldview of Islam.

Tawhid or Unity of the Creator

It is useful to start by positing that Islam, according to the Muslim understanding, is not a historical incident whose beginning is traced to the time of the Prophet Mohammad and the revelation of the *Quran* to him. Islam, which means peace as well as submission and surrender to the will of the Creator, began with the creation of the world. All that is created submit naturally to the Creator, and by their mere existence, declare His oneness. This is the essence of the fundamental principle of faith which states *"there is no god but God."* The Arabic term for this concept is *Tawhid* or Unity of the Creator. As corollaries to *Tawhid*, submission and surrender constitute the heart of the Islamic worldview, and the Muslim religion is founded upon them.

Tawhid, as W. Chittick (1996) explains, stands outside history; it is a universal truth and an inherent quality of the original disposition of humankind. Thus, *Tawhid* pertains to the nature of reality and the substance of human intelligence. Ontologically, the objective reality is governed by *Tawhid*. In epistemological terms, the human soul always already knows its Creator and is naturally disposed to behave in harmony with the laws governing the universe. Knowledge of the reality of the universe is latent within every soul, and the laws in the universe are informed by *Tawhid*. In other words, the Unity of the Creator governs everything.

Human understanding can, however, be different from reality. But this split between ontology and epistemology remains at the level of human understanding and its interactions with the manifestations of reality. The human soul and reality *per se* are fundamentally informed by *Tawhid*: reality, as manifested in the physical world, is governed by laws that all point to the one Creator, and the human soul is inherently ready and predisposed to know its Creator. Humankind, in the view of Islam, has been given reason to think and rationalize actions. Unlike all other creation, people have the freedom to choose their religion and the way they lead their lives. By the same token, Islam holds that each course of action leads to logical consequences for which an individual is responsible. Furthermore, Islam has outlined the right way to follow which will lead to harmony and balance. So each individual has the will to choose and the capability to do evil and good.

The *Tawhid*-based worldview has led Muslim scholars to pursue scientific research as leading essentially to the truth of religion. The *Quran* repeatedly calls humankind to contemplate its environment and the vast cosmos to know that its faith and belief system is in harmony with what is best for its primordial nature. In other words, the laws maintain for the universe its harmony and balance, and the belief system that religion calls for maintains for the human nature its balance and harmony.

Harmony in human systems is a necessary consequence of these laws and the belief system. These laws take the form of values and ethical principles that constitute good and acceptable behavior, which are conducive to the systemic good. These laws thus result in a social system marked by beauty and balance, both of which are facets of harmony. Consequently, these laws are the basis of an ethics and an aesthetics that guide one's process of becoming in the world.

For the Muslim scholars, throughout the history of Islam and up to our time, the study of the universe based on *Tawhid* led to the realization that since everything is created by God who is the Truth itself, then nothing in the universe can be without purpose or created in vain. Nothing created by the Truth (God) can be inherently false or purposeless. *"He created the heavens and the earth in true (proportions): He makes the night overlap the day, and the day overlap the night. He has subjected the sun and the moon (to His Law): each follows a course for a time appointed." (Quran, 39:5).*

Moreover, Muslim scholars studied the universe, as the macrocosm, without losing sight of the necessity to understand the human soul, the microcosm. For God has created this universe for the human being to be in it and act as His viceregent *khalifa*, as a trustee of the world. Thus, considering both the outer world and the inner emotional and spiritual life of the human being is essential. The ultimate goal of the entire scientific research enterprise for the Muslim scholars was, and still is, to come to peace with the purpose of creation, promote life, and contribute toward the establishment of civilization, to make the world a home-like place to live.

Consequently, the theory of knowledge in such a system does not separate scientific pursuits from the purposes of religion. *Tawhid* entails the unity of truth, and since there is only one truth, then there is no reason why science should oppose religion. Islam, in this sense, is anti-positivist, maintaining for humanity both its existential and spiritual nature. Scientific pursuits, put in the context of human systems dynamics, serve to promote the very purpose of creation, i.e. establish civilization for all human systems and promote the harmony of the entire eco-system.

Humanity's responsibility transcends immediate human systems out of which each person is an essential part. An individual's responsibility is wholistic in essence, and covers everything created: the birds in the sky, the fish in the oceans, the trees, and everything created. Civilization in this sense can be defined as the process of making life — in all systems whether human, natural, or animal — in harmony with the purpose of creation: to live in peace, and in submission to the will of the Creator, which is what the word Islam exactly means. So, to see complexity from the worldview of Islam is to engage in a project of establishing civilization for all existing systems. The pursuit of knowledge becomes an act of worship and a conscious process of *becoming* at home in the universe.

Causality

In the view of Islam, causes and their effects are all creations of God. This view is founded on the principle that the Creator is one. The history of Muslim philosophy, with its different schools of thought and orientations, had and still has one ultimate goal, to prove *(Tawhid)* or the Unity of the Divine Principle. The unity of the Creator leads to unity in all things created, and in their complex interrelationships, they all lead to the purpose of creation, and point to the one Creator upon whom their very existence depends. *"He is the Beginning and He is the End; He is the Outer Appearance and He the Inner Reality" (Quran, 57:3).*

Muslim scholars and philosophers all agree that only God causes everything, and there is nothing that happens without His knowledge and will. The Muslim scholar, Abu Hamid Al-Ghazali (d. 505H/1111G), describes causality and its implications. For Al-Ghazali, there is no necessary connection between external events. Only God causes everything. Consequently, there is no room for *secondary* causes. Through this argument, Al-Ghazali wants to affirm God's omnipotence. *"According to the Islamic view, Allah is the knower of all things and the cause of all events. His Knowledge, Power, and Unity overshadow the possibility of any secondary cause."*[1] According to Wolfson (1976), as quoted in Karen Harding (1994), Al Ghazali believed that *"ever since the creation of the world, whenever God creates certain events in succession to other events, He creates in men the knowledge or the impression that, barring miracles, the same events will continue to be created by Him in the future in the same order of succession."*[2] In Kantian terms, the mind derives its laws from the created nature; it does not impose its laws on nature.

For Al-Ghazali, objects endure over time not because of inherent properties that cause them to persist. Al-Ghazali builds his ontology on the premise of what he calls *"continuous creation"*: God creates things anew each moment. Thus, objects persist and continue to exist and interact not because of some inherent properties and causal laws, but because of God's continuous creative act in the world. Al-Ghazali's ontology is fundamentally different from the Newtonian mechanical worldview and similar in many ways to the non-Newtonian view of quantum theory. *"Both quantum theory and Al-Ghazali agree that objects do not possess inherent properties and independent existence. They both deny that the regularities in the behavior of objects be attributed to the existence of small laws. They also deny that events are completely predictable."*[3] Despite their similarities, the two philosophies have different frames of reference.

The Divine dynamic power of creation keeps change in space and time. Everything changes in such wisdom that it achieves its goals. However, the distinctive tenet of the Islamic worldview of causality is that the relation between the effects and the causes is not a necessary one. But the Creator, in His benevolence, has made this universe a home for the human species to live in and establish civilization for all existing systems, and to propagate the *systemic good* based on moral and ethical principles. *"It is He Who has made the earth manageable for you, to traverse through its tracts and enjoy of the sustenance which He furnishes, and unto Him is the resurrection."* (Quran, 67:15).

The rationality of the causal relations, resulting in a home-like universe, leads one to trust the Creator and therefore believe that effects will follow from causes, not in and of themselves, but as a result of the will of the Creator. *"As Al-Ghazali and Hume had found out despite their ideological differences, there is no necessity to any causal connection. Indeed, what we call causality is mere 'following upon' and repetition, leading us to believe that a cause is usually followed by its effects."*[4] As such, causality is a psychological habit resulting from our experiences through time. In this way, we are able to predict the usual behavior of phenomena in the universe.

Al-Ghazali maintains that the relationship between cause and effect is a composite relationship which involves an indefinite number of contributory factors. Even apparently simple phenomena are complex in that effects are hardly the result of a singular cause but of a plurality of causes. So it would be simplistic, therefore, to attribute a social action in a given human system to a single cause. Human systems are rather non-linear, and the thought process that sets to explicate them also needs to be so.

Al-Ghazali contends that reality, ontologically speaking, is not the result of simple relationships between observable effects and single causes. Non-material factors too play a role in the emergence of phenomena. Thus, epistemologically speaking, a person cannot claim to know all the causes of all the effects. He or she can however know some of the causes of given effects. This is best exemplified in the following Quranic verse: *"And with Him are the keys of the invisible. None but He knows them. And He knows what is in the land and the sea. Not a leaf falls, but He knows it, not a grain amid the darkness of the earth, naught of wet or dry but (it be noted) in a clear record' (Quran, 6:8).*

Purposefulness and Intentionality

For Muslim thinkers and philosophers, there is wisdom in everything created. The universe is rational and made homelike and livable for all created species. Rationality here means that there is a habit in creation that certain effects follow from certain causes. Habit of this sequence creates in an individual the habit of expecting effects to follow from causes. The worldview of Islam also tells each of us that, in addition, this habit is made possible because the Creator wants it to be so. Therefore rationality is not a mechanistic sequence, but a divinely guided one.

The rationality of creation implies order and purposefulness, for the Creator, *"being the Wise and the Rational creates things that must embody the quality of reason, which denotes order, purpose, and the truth."*[5]

The *Quran* insists that individuals pursue a *wholistic* understanding of creation. Everyone's purpose should be to live in harmony with the wisdom of creation, its purpose, his or her own position in this vast creation, and the purpose of his or her being here and now.

Islam, as a worldview, repeatedly invites the individual to reflect on the large cosmos as well as his or her inner world. The *Quran* refers to the first as *Afaq* (horizons in the physical world) and the second as *Anfus* (inner selves). *"Travel through the earth and see how Allah originated creation." (Quran, 29:20).* Both the cosmos and one's inner world are created by the same Creator. Both have a purpose. The cosmos is made subservient for humanity to establish civilization and promote peace. The cosmos readily puts itself at the disposal of humankind so each individual may achieve his or her purposes. The cosmos is governed by laws that sustain harmony and beauty. Humanity has been given laws and a belief system that guarantee for each person harmony, beauty, and an ethical life. Both the physical laws and the religious codes naturally match and give life harmony and purpose.

Our inner world is another equally vital source of knowledge leading to a more enlightened understanding of life. *"We will show them Our signs in the universe and in their own souls as well, until it becomes manifest to them that it is the truth." (Quran, 41:53). "Do they not reflect within themselves?" (Quran, 30:8).*

Out of a dual reflection on the cosmos outside and the inner world of the self, emerges a thought process that is wholistic and integrative, rather than linear and isolationistic. The emergence of this mindset has possibilities that each of us has the will and power to translate into the realm of actuality, for many contemplate the outside universe and within themselves and yet their thinking is trapped in mechanistic modes and processes. The wholistic mindset, in the realm of social life, considers both the self and the other as integral elements in the complex web of relations, the self with its history and aspirations and the other likewise. As such, the Islamic worldview is essentially wholistic and systemic — one that integrates rather than divides; one that concerns itself with complex patterns rather than simple single events. Unlike mainstream science, it does not dissect to understand.

Humanity is endowed with the capacity to transform creation so as to embody ethical and aesthetic patterns in harmony with the laws of nature and the laws of morality. Each of us is part of an infinite, complex web of relations with all creation. While one's being is a result of the act of creation in the first place, his or her becoming in the world is a process in motion toward the fulfillment of the systemic good, and the moral and ethical purpose of creation, i.e. civilization on earth. *"The truth is from your Lord, let him who will, believe and let him who will, disbelieve." (Quran, 18:29).* All individuals have the capacity to effect change in themselves and the world around them, in a very dynamic and interactive way. *"And there is nothing for man but what he strives for." (Quran, 39:53). "Truly Allah does not change that which is with a people until they change that which is within themselves." (Quran, 13:11).* Free will implies responsibility for the implications of one's actions on the entire system of which he or she is part. Thus, it is a systemic responsibility to the extent that, for instance, killing an innocent being is like killing the entire humanity *(Quran, 5:32).*

The cosmic order consists of rational laws. These laws permeate all aspects of reality, whether they are material, psychological, social or aesthetic, whether in the realm of human systems or in the animal kingdom. These laws all serve the moral and ethical purposes of creation itself. The One Creator sustains for these laws their consistency continuously. The act of creation is a dynamic process. It is continual and forever renewing until an appointed time that the Creator wills it to cease to be. It is dynamic as it allows unlimited realms of possibilities.

There is always already a purpose to everything in life. But the ultimate end to everything is the ultimate purpose of creation, i.e. every purpose is subject to other purposes until they all lead to the final purpose that ends in Allah. It is an individual's mission to maintain and continually foster an alignment between his or her pursuits and projects and the purpose of creation. The realm of possibilities for one's projects is limitless. The cosmos has been made greater than our scientific discoveries can ever encompass *"Assuredly the creation of the heavens and the earth is a greater (matter) than the creation of men: yet most men know not" (Quran, 40:57).*

As such, we are always in a position of challenge and search. But our search is not a haphazard search for the unknown but a purposeful search that leads to the systemic good, thus enhancing harmony by unearthing the beautiful and the good latent in the universe. The potential for evil is just as possible for each individual as is the potential for good. It is each person's free will to choose either way. But Islam calls for the systemic good and all that promotes peace and harmony and beauty.

Everyone's action thus has to be intentionally purposeful in the sense that it is not haphazard, and it points eventually to Allah and His purpose of creating life. *"That all things in creation serve a purpose and that all purposes are internalized as means and ends to one another makes the world one telic system, vibrant and alive, full of meaning. The birds in the sky, the stars in the firmament, the fishes in the depth of the ocean, the plants and the elements — all constitute integral parts of the system...Together, they make an organic body whose members and organs are interrelated..."*[6]

Purposefulness is facilitated through a dynamic, marked by harmony and concordance, between nature's laws and each person's being. Nature is made subservient to humankind, and the substance of this subservience is the complex network of relationships existing among everything alive in nature. Consequently, in the view of Islam, causality cannot be but with a purpose. Purposefulness is always already existent in the physical and natural systems, and in the animal kingdom. Humans are the only created beings who have the free will and the power to make a choice. Such a conception imparts meaning on every single action in life.

In the process of the complex, causal interrelationships, systems' agents self-organize and bring about emergent properties, which by virtue of the logic underlying the Islamic worldview, equally serve a purpose. Purposeful self-organization leads to meaningful emergent properties. Purposefulness results in coherence and purposeful self-organizing processes lead to emergent properties that work in alignment with the essential purpose of the interacting agents. In human systems, purpose guides the self-organizing processes, and meaningful emergence is the ultimate goal. The possibilities of what shape or magnitude, or what time the outcome occurs, are limitless.

Purposeful emergence in nature also derives its meaning from the affinity between the truth, reason, and reality. Any occurrence in nature reflects this affinity. Possibilities of contradiction are impossible. It is emergence with wisdom and guidance. So it is guided emergence that maintains for the ecosystem balance and harmony. *"Reflect on the Divine mercy as revealed in the growing of provisions, vegetables, grains and fruits, gradually emerging in a slow succession. It is a blessing that they do not grow all at the same time, for if they were to grow like this on land, or if they did not grow on branches and stalks, much harm would take place, and many benefits that accrue from their emerging gradually would be missed…[E]ach season is so for the benefits of plants that are precisely adapted to it."*[7]

This affinity is further harmonized with the Divine Revelation, as indicated in the script, i.e. the *Quran*. Thus the closed book proves the veracity of the laws existing in the open book, nature. Natural laws in turn prove the truth of the principle laid out in the script. *"This logical equivalence of reason, truth and reality with the fact of Revelation is the most critical principle that epistemology has ever known."*[8]

Purposeful self-organization and meaningful emergence in human systems, in the Islamic worldview, take effect when one's actions are in coherence with the cosmic purpose entrusted to humankind: to promote life and development, and thus to build civilization. This development process cannot be left to blind chance or difference of opinion for the sake of individual freedom. This is not to say that the emergent properties are known before the self-organizing process actually takes place. While the exact shape and final form of emergence is unknowable, purpose and intentionality guide the process within a limitless realm of possibilities and potentialities.

The selfness in self-organization, in the Islamic sense, is such that it always obeys the unity of truth. Self-organization is always already confined within the boundaries of the unity of truth. Self-organization is not in any sense a free, haphazard process, resulting in blind unpredictable patterns. Selfness in self-organization is a bounded selfness, yet in a limitless space of creative possibilities.

So for Islam, creation, and therefore life, is meant to be. It is not accidental nor a result of some blind meaningless "soup of life." Furthermore, life is not evil or bad, nor is an individual asked to seek redemption for some original sin or to exercise self-denial to live outside history. In human systems, there are processes that take shape through human free will. Islam stipulates that these processes enact morality in co-existence with the laws of nature. This enactment occurs in the context of complex networks of relations and events in the empirical world.

A human being is the only created agent capable of enacting these moral laws at will. When one chooses to build a civilization based on these moral and ethical ideals, the human race lives in harmony with the laws of nature; he or she learns from its processes and designs his or her artifacts, models, and paradigms to sustain that harmony. When individuals choose to craft moral laws in accordance with their own wishes, they are at odds with the very laws governing nature. They conjure up false images of life and live accordingly.

So for Islam, the Creator knows what best fits the cosmos as natural laws, and what best suits human nature as moral laws. *'Do they want some other code than God's though each and every thing in heaven or earth is under His sway? And all will be led back towards God' (Quran, 3:83).*

People are free to enact those moral laws or craft new ones. Each individual's physical structure, psychological disposition, the natural environment around him or her, are all subservient to his or her choices. In both cases, a person is making history come alive. He or she is enjoined to live up to the values and morals in harmony with the very purpose of creation, to design the self-organizing processes and their emergents in the individual's life and align them to the grand nobler life purposes. When one chooses to be at home in the universe, at home with its embedded laws, at home with the moral laws that a *priori* co-exist with the natural laws, then one is playing the role of the agent, free as it were, that facilitates the Creator's purposes to enter history and become real. *"Man is therefore a cosmic bridge between the higher echelons of the Divine Will and historical reality. Evidently his being is of tremendous significance."*[9]

So significant is one's being, in the view of Islam, that it would be futile to turn his or her life into an aimless project, a process that is subject to its own dynamics and influenced by its environment. Every human being is significant because every action he or she performs in the universe is intricately connected to a grand network of meaning and purpose. Purpose adds perspective and quality to one's being as he or she moves in time and space. As such, being in the position of the Creator's viceregent on earth, each of us is expected to *"transform creation into the divine patterns, i.e. to rearrange its materials so as to make them fully and beneficially subserve human needs, the material…as well as the moral. […] In the very act of transforming creation, humans ought to instantiate the ethical values by choosing to enter into those acts of transformation in an ethical way."* [10]

It is useful to add here that this view is not in any way consistent with a mechanistic, causal, and Newtonian worldview, where ends are known and predetermined. This view sets the simple rules for human systems and leaves the complexity dynamics, i.e. self-organization and emergence, for each person to design. Natural systems self-organize in accordance with rules that are best fit for them to maintain balance and harmony for the entire eco-system. Animals behave while guided by their instincts; they self-organize and the emergent patterns contribute to the harmony of the eco-system. For human systems, the Creator has set simple rules that are essentially in harmony with the other existing systems. Simple rules in the form of values and ethical systems that serve as signposts for guidance. All are urged to contemplate nature and learn from the complexities of natural systems and what it leads to. What else can they learn except that everything around them is engaged in sustaining balance and order.

In their own systems, they are required to work by the simple rules and appreciate the complexity without losing sight of the intent of the simple rules.

Thus the whole drive of creation is to establish civilization for the benefit of all species, on the basis of a value system which is essentially in harmony with the natural laws governing creation. For the human species, this constitutes the core of the human identity and real value. Amidst the diversity of human species, in race or color or otherwise, what makes a person or a nation more worthy is the extent to which they assume their responsibility for the systemic good, beyond the different characteristics that remain accidental to their true identity.

Amidst the complexity of one's undertakings, the inner core of each person's existence should drive his or her projects and engineer the results — cultural artifacts, social organizations — that come from the countless non-linear, self-organizing processes in his or her life.

A Muslim worldview is not limited in scope and methodology to reality as it is; it looks farther to what reality ought to be, and says that all energy should be channeled to achieve that purpose. Nature is already always engaged in that purposeful process. Human knowledge cannot, in an Islamic sense, establish its concepts and methodologies in researching human reality *"in abstraction from what that reality ought to be. Any investigation of a human 'is' must therefore include its standing as an 'ought to be' within the realm of ends..."*[11]

Natural laws reveal the pattern by which the Creator manages the cosmos. Moral laws, by which we are to lead our lives, ought to actualize the Creator's divine pattern in human affairs. The complex self-organizing processes permeating human life should not be left to yield results contrary to the divine patterns that human life ought to live by. Otherwise life itself becomes meaningless. Human life patterns become incongruous with nature's patterns. Self-organizing processes should be channeled, with vibrant energy, toward the greater, systemic good. Thus, each person's creative engagement is in harmony with God's creationist will.

On Predictability

In a complex system, based on the concept of continuous creation, it is beyond our power to predict the outcome of interactions in human systems. All we can do is to deal with the simple rules of ethics based on the value system, and trust that the complex unfolds with potentialities that may suit our needs one way or the other. For example, offer your morning prayers at dawn in congregation and leave the unfolding of the day to the dynamics of the known habits of life laws and the unknown surprises that only God facilitates for you, to your utmost surprise in many instances.

It is in the habit of things that effects follow from causes. It is possible, however, that God wants otherwise and thus the outcome is delayed in time or may take the form of an event or set of events that are not as expected. The resulting human characteristic or competency, thus developed and nurtured, is one of trust that even the seemingly unwanted results have their wisdom. Good results may be delayed for a good reason such as for self-development, emotional intelligence, and intellectual maturity. Allah is also named *Rabb, "one who rears, fosters, or nourishes, as a caretaker who gradually helps nurture something or someone to a state of completion, maturity, or independence."* [12]

These are some of the fundaments that make up the way a Muslim mind works. This mindset is essentially holistic and able to appreciate naturally the complexity of life. A Newtonian explanation of the world is *a priori* alien to this mindset.

On The Power of Small Things

The butterfly is entrusted, through its *Fitra* (primordial nature), to flap its wings, creating all kinds of effects unseen to the eye. The butterfly does not need to think to create the effects; the purposeful laws inherent in the universe take care of the rest. The butterfly has an inherent vision that takes its content from its *Fitra*. In our human systems, we are like butterflies. Conscious as we are, we have the power to design the effects of our actions. We may not know when, where, or what the particular effects may be.

How many times did we find ourselves in a situation where we surprisingly got the help we most needed even without asking for it? We wonder how and why.

There are silent effects in action that come as a result of previous actions. The feedback loop, or the cycle, reaches its maturity only within a specific time frame. You have done something good, and you think it has passed into oblivion, buried in time's unforgiving womb. However, the dynamic of silent effects in action, through feedback loops, has its own ways.

The habits of events, influenced by the specific environments in which they occur, usually lead to the expected and desired results. Unexpected factors, however, may come into the picture and drive the process to undesired results. These factors could well be in themselves results of earlier situations not addressed properly that have been latent within the system until such time as they emerge.

The complexity of causal interconnectedness, both as causes and effects, is governed by a beautiful and wise system of proportion and measure: *"Verily, all things have We created in proportion and measure." (Quran, 54:49).*

Every act, small or large, has its fullest consequences according to a just and fair measure. The sub-systems operate at their local levels, yet their ripple effects travel throughout the system. The entire system echoes back albeit in varying degrees. In dealing with the others, one is enjoined not to undermine the effect and the importance of even the slightest act. The Prophet gives the example of smiling in the face of all those around you. However insignificant and small it may be as a social act, its effects on the entire community are immeasurable. It is that beautiful system of measure that takes up the obvious and latent effects and leads them to their destinations in accordance with the overall purpose of each local system. It is a feedback loop at work; we tend to see the beginning part of the loop, and because of time trajectories, which tend to be longer that we can appreciate; we tend to forget about the end of the loop. Meanwhile, the latent laws are at work. To echo Al-Ghazali, time has imprinted in our psyche the habit of expecting the obvious results from the obvious causes. The result is a linear thought process. Causes have no power in themselves to produce effects. Therefore, we have to keep in touch with the Primary Cause of all effects. One way to realize that, for the sake of a harmonious dynamics for a better human civilization, is through the essential values and ethics that He has ordained for us, and which are essentially always already in harmony with the laws of nature, and in concordance with our human nature. The result is a complete affinity between our acts, our human nature, and nature. We will be, as it were, at home in the universe.

Fouad Mimouni

Fouad Mimouni is currently the Head of Training and Development in a multinational Islamic Development organization. He is also managing the Executive Development Program and the Young Professionals Program of the same organization. He received his BA from Morocco in English linguistics in 1997. He was a Fulbright scholar at Indiana University where he received his MA in contemporary critical theories in 1990. He is now finishing his doctorate at Hull University in the application of complexity theory in organizations.

His areas of interest include systems thinking, complexity theory, emotional intelligence, and coaching. He is also conducting research on the implications of complexity theory on human systems when viewed from different worldviews. He can be contacted at: fmimouni26@hotmail.com.

Notes

1. Seyyed H. Nasr. *Islamic Life and Thought.* Albany: State University of New York Press, 1981, p.92.

2. Karen Harding. "Causality Then and Now: Al Ghazali and Quantum Theory." *American Journal of Islamic Social Sciences* 10:2, (1994), p.168.

3. Yamine B. Mermer. *Induction, Science and Causation: Some Critical Reflections.* Islamabad: Islamic Research Institute,1996, p. 15.

4. Isma'il Raji Al-Faruqi. *Meta-Religion: A Framework For Islamic Moral Theology.* Washington: Islamic Institute for Strategic Studies. Policy Paper No. 5, June 2000, p. 77.

5. Khalifa Abdul Hakim, *Islamic Ideology: The Fundamental Beliefs and Principles of Islam and their Application to Political Life.* Lahore: Institute of Islamic Culture, 1993, p. 28.

6. Al-Faruqi, op. cit., p. 78.

7. Anas Abdul-Hameed Al-Qoz, *Men and the Universe: Reflections of Ibn Al-Qayyem.* Riyadh: Darussalam, 2000, p. 306.

8. Al-Faruqi, op. cit., p. 83.

9. Ibid., p. 86.

10. Ibid., p. 88.

11. Ibid., p. 102.

12. Ahmad Z. Hammad, *The Opening to The Quran.* Illinois: Quranic Literacy Institute, 1996, p. 43.

FROM THE BUREAUCRACY IN JUNEAU, THE TASK SEEMED QUITE SIMPLE: DESIGN AND IMPLEMENT A TRAINING PROGRAM FOR CHILD CARE WORKERS ACROSS THE STATE. AS THE CREATOR AND COORDINATOR OF THE PROJECT, SUE POPE SAW SOMETHING QUITE DIFFERENT AND MUCH MORE COMPLEX. DIVERGENT AGENDAS OF INDIVIDUAL CHILDREN AND WORKERS, AGENCIES, FUNDING STREAMS, AND STATE POLICY MAKERS CREATED MASSIVELY ENTANGLED OBJECTIVES. GEOGRAPHICAL, CULTURAL, AND HISTORICAL DIVISIONS DISRUPTED COOPERATION AND SHARED ACTION. CONSTRAINTS ON TIME AND MONEY RESTRICTED THE ABILITY TO BUILD COMMUNICATIONS AMONG PLAYERS IN THE SYSTEM. IN THIS UNCOUPLED AND OUT-OF-CONTROL LANDSCAPE, SUE SAW OPPORTUNITY. SHE WAS ABLE TO USE HER EMERGING PERSONAL THEORIES ABOUT COMPLEXITY TO ESTABLISH AN ADAPTIVE NETWORK. BY ATTENDING TO THE COMPLEX DYNAMICS, SHE WAS ABLE TO SET CONDITIONS FOR A SELF-ORGANIZING PROCESS THAT CONTINUES TO INCREASE THE COHERENCE AND CAPACITY OF THE WHOLE.

Trying to Stay Afloat in Alaska

By Susan M. Pope, Ph.D.

The Landscape

Vast distances. Few roads. Sparse population. Isolated communities. More child abuse, Fetal Alcohol Spectrum Disorders, and suicide than anywhere else in the nation. More oil production and revenue than anywhere else in the nation. Emerging tribal self-determination and economic clout. Intense competition for skilled workers. Fierce battles over natural resources. Stubborn independence, hope, and optimism.

This is the landscape I traverse daily in my work with the Alaska Association of Homes for Children, an organization representing 20 non-profit children's residential facilities across the state. My role is to assess, create, and implement training programs for the staffs of these agencies. But the job is much more and much less than these tasks.

I am a trail builder, creating paths between and among the agencies as well as the political, economic, and social systems through which they must travel. At first, I did not know this is what I had to do. I ran in circles on well-trod paths before I created new ones. Gradually I discovered these simple rules: narrow winding trails may lead to hidden gems; if you are low on resources near-by destinations are worth achieving; and if invited, all kinds of people are willing to walk with you. In short, viewing my project as *a complex adaptive system*—a collection of constantly changing people and organizations relating to each other in unpredictable ways—helps me retain my sanity and locate patterns that indicate small but significant progress toward improving the quality of care for children.

Background

Three years ago I left a secure, well-paying job in a large bureaucracy with a generous retirement plan to take on a brand-new program with no staff, little money, and huge potential. Professionally, I had come full-circle. I began my career in human services over 25 years ago, working as a family therapist for one of the agencies in the new project. Since then I had meandered through private counseling practice, corporate training, public education, and now back again to social services. In my journey, I discovered I do not do well in large traditional systems that avoid innovation.

Now, my job is to identify the common training needs among the 20 agencies spanning the state — from Barrow to Ketchikan (a distance covering roughly one-fifth of the continental U.S.) — and create a curriculum and delivery system to meet those needs. The agencies varied in size and purpose from small emergency shelters to large long-term adolescent treatment facilities. All were desperate for ways to train their inexperienced staff to deal with some of most challenging children in the child protection and juvenile justice systems. In addition, they hoped that better training would help them reduce the staff turnover that frequently reached 100% a year.

But there was more to the project. The Division of Family and Youth Services, which was funding the project, had its own agenda. It wanted to improve the quality of care for the children in custody, to decrease the number of referrals that the agencies declined, and to bring back the children to the state who were being sent elsewhere for treatment. As the only staff member in the project I was to dance between the sometimes-competing agendas of my two constituencies.

A Small but Significant Shift Leads to a Marriage of Convenience

Even though I had studied complex systems theory in graduate school, at first I failed to recognize its application to this project. In my haste to make up for lost time—I was hired halfway through the first grant year—I viewed my task from a traditional problem-solving model: identify needs, build a curriculum, train trainers, create capacity in agencies and communities, reduce turnover, improve treatment of children, evaluate impact, make everyone happy. Quickly I recognized that the agencies, funding streams, political and economic environments, and players changed so quickly that a traditional model of planning, goal setting, and evaluation would not work at all. Change was the only constant in the system. Trainers quit shortly after completing their training; agencies lacked funding for staff coverage to attend training. Two member agencies closed their doors amid internal controversy. The state changed its system of paying for placement.

The Alaska Association of Homes for Children (AAHC) was created 15 years ago to form a single voice to advocate for more funds for children's residential facilities. Before joining forces in the AAHC, agencies negotiated rates individually with the state Division of Family and Youth Services (DFYS). "Deals" were made and, according to long-time AAHC members, some agencies were paid more than others for delivering the same services. So, AAHC was born out of an effort to equalize funding and present a "united front," to DFYS and the state legislature. This history reveals the adversarial nature of the relationship that shaped the landscape in which I worked.

Funding for my training and development project resulted from several years of complaints from AAHC members that they had no resources to train their staffs. In a typical scenario, the state would request placement for a child who had been removed from his or her home or foster home. The local agency would accept the child. Sooner or later, the young person would "do something" to get rejected from the placement. The residential agency would complain that the child's behavior was too severe for their facility and turn the child away. The social worker searched for another placement, usually in another community. Most agencies had no full-time trainers. Smaller agencies in rural communities (some with no more than five beds and seven staff) hired local people with only high school educations or GED's. These individuals may have had successful experiences in raising their own children, but were ill-equipped to deal with the traumatized children who entered residential care. In many communities, a large percentage of children in care were fetal-alcohol affected. So, with an administration in Juneau (our state capital) whose cornerstone commitment was to children's welfare, the state agreed to provide a small amount of money to AAHC to launch a staff training program. A new, collaborative partnership between the state and the Association was consummated.

This complex and dynamic environment demonstrates many of the patterns that are characteristic of complex systems and human systems dynamics, including:

- Change through connection
- Sensitivity to initial conditions
- Emerging goals
- Adapting to uncertainty

- Amplifying difference

- Discovering self-similarity

- Redefining success as fit with environment

I will describe how I discovered each of these patterns throughout the evolution of the project.

Change Through Connections: The "Ah-ha" Experience

At the end of year one of the project I was ready to quit. We had established a basic curriculum for residential staff and it was being delivered by trainers in various agencies. But half of our trainers had quit, and my yearly needs assessment had uncovered a deeper and broader training agenda that I could see no way of meeting. Armed with a newly devoured copy of Olson and Eoyang's book (2001) and fresh from a workshop with the authors at the OD Network conference, I realized that although I saw the complexity in the systems in which I was operating, I was acting as if I was in a traditional stable environment. I lacked a true connection to the other agents in my system and we lacked a connection to a larger purpose. I had never asked my constituents what they meant by "quality" care for children or how they would define success. So, in the final month of the first year of the project, I convened the first face-to-face meeting of my advisory committee and people from the state juvenile justice and child protection systems.

Through the course of our day-long conversations a shift occurred in the group and in me. We came to see that we that we shared a common understanding of what we meant by quality of care for children. By the end of the day we agreed on a core purpose and values for the project and the core competencies and goals we wished to achieve. Although the individuals in this group never again assembled face-to-face, I still feel we are connected and working to create common changes in our respective systems. At that point, I recognized that the project had taken on the characteristics of a complex adaptive system, and although we couldn't predict the outcomes, we each had similar intentions for change. The connections we established that day proved to be fertile seeds that took root and grew later in the project.

The Importance of Initial Conditions

From its birth, the project "floated" semi-autonomously among governmental and not-for-profit systems — everyone's child yet no one's child. This was not a planned decision, but emerged out of expediency. Initial decisions regarding who claimed the project, who would be hired, and where the project coordinator would be housed all contributed toward the later success of the project as a malleable container for exchanges of information and expertise.

When DFYS initially scraped together the funding to begin our project the Association (AAHC) could not receive money because, while it is a professional organization it is not incorporated as a formal not-for-profit organization. Who would accept the money? One agency in the Association would have to add statewide responsibility to its already-full local human service agenda.

A group of AAHC member representatives huddled to discuss who should shoulder the additional money and responsibilities. Historically, battles for resources pit urban and rural Alaskan communities against each other. Urban areas such as Anchorage and Fairbanks are seen by rural communities and villages as resource-rich and insensitive to the needs and issues of smaller, more isolated communities. Life Quest, a comprehensive mental health center with several programs operating in the Matanuska-Susitna Valley, about 50 miles north of Anchorage, offered to administer the grant. This solved the urban-rural dilemma. Wasilla, the home office of Life Quest, was more rural than urban, yet still on the road system and positioned centrally in the state. As principal of the program, I would report directly to the CEO of Life Quest. Unlike most other agencies in AAHC, Life Quest offers a wide array of mental health services to an age span of consumers stretching from birth to death. Their children's group home is just a small component of their whole organization.

The physical location of my office also provided me with opportunities to weave connections among agents who would not ordinarily form relationships. Since Life Quest had limited office space, and I live in Anchorage, the University of Alaska Anchorage School of Social Work offered in-kind office space for the project in their Family and Youth Services Training Academy, located off the main campus in Anchorage. The Academy provides training to all child protection workers in the state. This connection has proven invaluable in terms of access to resources, building relationships across traditional adversaries, and most importantly, providing a container for diverse agents who work with children (child protection workers, foster parents, and residential workers) to come together to learn.

Finally, the decision to hire me, on the second round of recruitment, influenced the future shape of the project. I am an inside/outsider. Although early in my career, I worked for one of the AAHC agencies, I worked in the outpatient component. I have never worked in a children's residential facility. I have extensive experience in program management and training design and delivery, however. This meant that I entered the project without allegiances to particular residential treatment models and curious to learn what worked. I was also outside the political arenas in which the other agents were immersed. So, I arrived on the scene naïve, optimistic, grateful for autonomy, eager to learn, and without preconceived outcomes.

Emerging Goals And Adapting to Uncertainty

At the same time we were holding our face-to-face dialogue session at the end of the first year, our political landscape quaked and shifted again. The state changed its funding requirements for children placed in residential care. (DFYS was trying to capture more of the Medicaid funding that was allocated to children in care.) Instead of flat rates for available beds they would be paid for actual occupancy. In addition, the state placed new educational requirements on the agencies. A percentage of staff (depending on "level of care" provided by the agency) was required to have bachelor's degrees or complete the curriculum we had developed. Some agencies, mostly small rural ones, would benefit financially from this new arrangement, but would have trouble fulfilling the educational requirements. Other agencies, mostly larger urban agencies, could easily meet the educational requirements but would lose money because they had been receiving direct Medicaid funding. Again, this divided the ranks of the AAHC. In addition, DFYS added a new requirement that the agencies would have two years to become accredited. DFYS, in turn, was under its own pressure to "look good" as they prepared for the first federal review of their child protection system. The regular fall meeting between AAHC and DFYS boiled with hostile debate.

In this environment I struggled with three questions regarding our tiny project:

1. How do I survive in the midst of the competition among all of the agents in the systems?

2. How do we define success?

3. How do we measure it?

A visit from Glenda Eoyang to the University of Alaska Anchorage's complex systems group provided a welcome perspective. She shared with me three insights that still shape my leadership of the project. They were: think quality instead of quantity in evaluating the project; see competition as an opportunity to adapt; and seek out differences that make a difference.

Since then, although I still play the numbers game with my grant administrators in Juneau, I focus on quality as defined by building agency capacity in three core competencies developed in our face-to-face dialogue at the end of the first year. These serve as my simple rules. They are:

1. Build healthy relationships (with children in care).

2. Understand child development.

3. Create a positive treatment environment.

Other goals have emerged or have fallen away in response to how they contribute to carrying these out. One goal with unexpected impact emerged out of a pattern created by allocation of grant funds to pay for staff travel. This proved to be a "difference which makes a difference."

Funding for staff travel provided rare and valuable opportunities for agencies to share information and learn from each other. Since we are a state with limited road access, air travel from one community to another frequently costs as much as a trip to New York or Europe. Originally, I intended to devote travel funds to local and regional training, building capacity in geographic regions. I soon discovered that, with Anchorage as the travel hub of the state, it was cheaper to fund a training session in Anchorage than pay for people to travel within their region. This meant that staff from the whole state converged in one training session. This yielded valuable exchanges of program information. As the participants shared information they discovered each other's expertise and began requesting funds to "import" other staff to their agency to provide training and program consultation. When the CEO's of the agencies discovered that travel funding was available they began requesting program consultation from their AAHC peers whose program knowledge they respected. What started as a few shifts in budget categories, emerged into a "consultation and technical assistance" goal for this year's grant cycle.

Because I viewed the entire project from a "learning" rather than "training" perspective I encouraged agencies and DFYS to use me as a conduit for knowledge exchanges. Soon, I was getting calls from DFYS requesting suggestions on which staff from "strong" agencies could assist those which were struggling. After several informal exchanges, I created a "learning contract" between the requesting and consulting parties so we could capture the learning and share it with others as appropriate.

Recognizing and supporting these emerging patterns contributes to agency capacity-building in other ways I will spell out below. With a change in governor and administration last fall, and an impending budget decrease, we face further opportunities to adapt.

Amplifying Differences and Discovering Self-Similarity

The third year of our project draws to a close. Has the momentum accelerated dramatically or am I just getting more astute at recognizing patterns? Probably both. Hiring a highly competent assistant last fall allowed me to stand back from the details, take a breath, and see the landscape more clearly. In addition, early decisions to invest in "differences which make a difference" are now revealing some sharp contrasts in quality. The most valuable of these investments has been in relationships with people.

One of the wisest decisions made by DFYS was to recruit a highly experienced program administrator away from one of the largest residential agencies in the state. For the past two years she has been in charge of program quality for residential children's facilities around the state. She is currently the administrator of our grant. I rely on her hands-on knowledge of effective program structure and management. She relies on my knowledge of trainers and learning resources. We both have the same goal—program quality. She travels to each agency, gaining an intimate knowledge of their strengths and weaknesses. Frequently, she calls on me to help strategize training and consultation options to assist struggling agencies. This collaboration both amplifies differences across the systems at the same time as it reveals self-similarity and coherence. Let me explain.

This year agencies have withered, re-structured, or diversified in response to the increased scrutiny by DFYS, shift in funding, changing administration *and perhaps* a more widely shared understanding of what makes a quality program. One of our goals this grant year was to conduct a literature review to reveal "what makes an effective residential treatment environment." With the help of a graduate student, we scoured the scant literature on the topic and produced a short summary with a bibliography, and circulated it to our funding source and constituents. What we found was that there was no *one model* of care that was better than others. But there were common elements of success including, a "family-like" atmosphere; involvement of family and community in treatment; coherent and predictable structure, positive nurturing relationships with adults, and building upon strengths of the youths and their families.

Another Ah-ha!

These small, common sense revelations illuminated the differences between the successful programs and the ones who were struggling. Two agencies led the others in terms of expertise and staff experience. Their staff was requested for consultation and training most frequently. Although they each had completely different treatment models, they all contained the elements of success revealed in our literature review. So, without knowing the outcomes, I was funneling resources into the systems that would most influence the other systems positively. This investment in resources, combined with the role of the DFYS quality expert, and the pressure to achieve accreditation has resulted in more program coherence across the agencies.

The same factors amplified the inadequacies of some programs that could not adapt to the environmental changes. One program has been taken over by another; one closed down to be reborn in the same community under a different organization; others have obtained funding outside the DFYS system.

"They" Are "Us"

I return to one of the "initial conditions" described in the beginning of this exploration—the importance of the project being physically located at the University of Alaska Family and Youth Services Training Academy. There are two reasons why this relationship has been essential to the success of the process. First, the director of the academy is what Galdwell (2000) calls a "Connector," a person with an incredible array of friends and acquaintances across the political, social, economic, and geographic spectrum; a person who delights in bringing people together. Second, while the purpose of the academy is to train the DFYS workforce it is a semi-autonomous unit belonging to the University of Alaska School of Social Work. Like my project, the Academy is an inside/outsider. These two factors have allowed us to ignore traditional boundaries between systems and collaborate on developing and delivering courses to combined audiences of residential staff, child protection workers, and foster parents. Tossing these three groups together into a common pool of knowledge washes away their distrust of each other. They gain a better appreciation and understanding of their respective roles and discover they do share a common desire to help children. Just the simple combination of quality curriculum, a trained facilitator, interested participants, and money to get them there, provides a container to develop coherence of purpose across systems. Now, in anticipation of reduction in travel funds, we are developing web-based courses open to the same participants.

Re-defining Success as Fit with the Landscape

It is June in Alaska. Here in Anchorage it is barely dusk at midnight. In Barrow at the children's emergency shelter the sun shines like a bare light bulb all night long. It still rains in Ketchikan, where mold might grow inside your shoes. I prepare my end of the year report. Today I meet face-to-face and via audio conference with representatives from two agencies who recently used grant funds to attend a conference on "Best Practices in Behavior Management" in Los Angeles sponsored by the Child Welfare League of America. They each have different ideas about how to use the information they collected in their agencies and their respective communities. The program manager from the rural community wants to help her staff do a better job at family assessment. The two representatives from the large urban organization want to explore using what they learned to develop a training program for managers in their community. Again, I'm clearing the trail to help them reach their individual destinations, in their very different terrains. In addition, I will be asking them to identify presenters from the conference who could address needs of other agencies in our Association. I am envisioning a "gathering" of agencies in the fall. As I take a few moments to mentally climb a hillside and survey the landscape of this project, I notice that my own role as a leader has gradually subsided. The project seems to be rolling forward with its own momentum. How do I measure success?

I consider the original agendas for the grant, from the agencies, and from DFYS. Have we reduced staff turnover in the agencies? I don't know. Have we decreased the number of children who are rejected or ejected from placement by the agencies? I don't know this either. Are fewer children placed outside the state for treatment? I don't know that either, although, several out-of-state organizations are exploring the viability of opening facilities in Alaska. What I do know is that the exchanges of knowledge and talent facilitated by this small project have helped build capacity in agencies ready to make use of them. A few agencies closed or lost programs because they could not adapt to the changes in funding, increased scrutiny, and pressure for greater quality. But other agencies organized to fill the vacated niches. An Anchorage agency tests out their own training "institute," a long-range goal whose time may be right. With an infusion of support and training from this grant, they move more quickly toward that goal, and may be ready to take over this project in another year.

How do I define success personally? Some days I can see no progress. But other days I believe I have cleared the path so that the people who care for children might travel an easier route. I have succeeded in connecting people with each other and with information. I think I have influenced the child welfare system in Alaska in some small way I will not ever know. Along the way I have learned much and formed rewarding relationships. Over the next few months I will ease out of this project. A new research project beckons, giving voice to the experiences of adults who lived in residential or foster care when they were children. I look forward to exploring this new landscape.

Susan M. Pope, Ph.D.
Sue Pope directs the Residential Provider Training Project of Life Quest Comprehensive Mental Health Services in Wasilla, Alaska. She earned her doctorate in Human and Organizational Development from The Fielding Institute. Her graduate studies focused on the transformational learning

experiences of working class women who were first in their families to complete higher education. She has a Master's Degree in Counseling Psychology, and a Bachelor's Degree in Journalism. In addition to developing curriculum and training for the staff of 20 non-profit children's residential agencies across Alaska, she conducts a coaching and consulting practice in Anchorage, Alaska. Sue's career background also includes freelance writing, family counseling, managing a corporate training department, and coordinating staff development for a large educational institution. She enjoys hiking, rafting, kayaking, and exploring wild places in Alaska and other far corners of the world. She also spends time learning important lessons about life from her grandchildren and volunteering with Healing Racism of Anchorage, an organization devoted to promoting cultural understanding and acceptance in her community.

BRENDA ZIMMERMAN AND BRYAN HAYDAY SHARE A POWERFUL TOOL FOR BUILDING AND MAINTAINING GENERATIVE RELATIONSHIPS WITHIN AND BETWEEN GROUPS. DERIVED FROM THEIR RESEARCH IN COMPLEX SYSTEMS AND FROM YEARS OF SUCCESSFUL CONSULTATION PRACTICE, THE TOOL REFLECTS SOME OF THE MOST CHALLENGING AND DISRUPTIVE FACETS OF GROUP DYNAMICS. AS A MIRROR, THE TOOL ALLOWS GROUPS TO ARTICULATE AND RESPOND TO UNSEEN DYNAMICS THAT BLOCK THEIR ABILITY TO WORK TOGETHER TOWARD COMMON ENDS. THE EXAMPLES ZIMMERMAN AND HAYDAY SHARE HELP DEMONSTRATE WHEN AND HOW THE TOOL WILL SUPPORT MANY KINDS OF GROUP DYNAMICS.

GENERATIVE RELATIONSHIPS STAR

Brenda J. Zimmerman, Ph.D.
Bryan C. Hayday

Complex Contexts Call for Relationships that Can Generate Novel Solutions

A generative relationship "produces new sources of value which cannot be foreseen in advance." (Lane and Maxfield, 1996, pg. 215).

There are two key components to this definition. The first is that the relationship produces something, which one of the members of the relationship could not have produced alone. Second, the source of value (whether it be a new product, service, form of distribution, or idea) could not have been foreseen in advance. It was created by the interaction between the parties.

Joint ventures may or may not be generative relationships. Often, they are merely partners who know what needs to be done *a priori* but each has a gap or deficiency that can be addressed by the other joint venture partner(s). Although this satisfies the first criterion of generative relationships, the source of value was foreseen in advance.

In complex contexts, where the future is inherently unknowable because the industry, sector, or society is going through transformational change, generative relationships are important. They allow the parties to learn as they co-create a new product, service, distribution process, or solution.

Generative relationships have the capacity to deal with complex contexts where change is happening both at the level of structure (e.g., who the players in the industry are) and at a conceptual level (e.g., the definitions of the product or service). The story of ROLM and the PBX (internal telephone systems) is an example of how quickly a whole industry can shift when a product is reconceived as a voice-interface management tool rather than a "telephone." Suddenly, computer manufacturers were key competitors with telephone giants like AT&T. ROLM fostered generative relationships to thrive in this environment, which they co-created.

How do you know whether a relationship will be generative or not? How do you enhance the generative potential of existing relationships? In an action research project with a non-profit social service agency, which struggled with this concept, we used a four pointed star to demonstrate the dimensions of a generative relationship. We used the acronym of STAR to make the idea memorable. Before looking at organizational examples of the STAR's use, we will define and describe the acronym with suggestions for practical applications.

Relationships with more generative potential are seen to have longer points on the generative relationship STAR. Each point of the STAR represents one key aspect of generative relationships and is a continuum from very low to very high levels of this aspect or attribute of a generative relationship.

Each point of the STAR represents one key aspect of generative relationships.

- Separateness or differences. There need to be differences in the background, skills, perspectives, or training of the parties. If all of the parties are similar, they may enjoy heated debates but may leave untouched or unchallenged the assumptions upon which both sides of the argument are based. One cannot challenge an assumption which goes unnoticed. Differences allow the partners or group to see things from a different perspective. They allow "facts" to be seen as "interpretations."

- Tuning (talking and listening). There need to be real opportunities to talk and listen to each other, to "tune" to the differences, with permission to challenge the status quo, sacred cows, or implicit assumptions of the context. The conceptual changes in a complex context can be profound. Opportunities for reflection allow the parties to grow and learn.

- Action opportunities. Talk is great but unless it is accompanied by acting on the talk, new sources of value will not be created. The parties need to be able to act together to co-create something new.

- Reason to work together. The parties need to have a reason to share resources and ideas, or to act as allies even if only for a short period. There has to be some mutual benefit to being aligned in a project. If the parties do not see value in working together, if they see each other as adversaries only rather than as allies for this piece of work, it is highly unlikely that they will co-create something of substantial value. They may talk and learn from each other, but then do the work of creating something new alone.

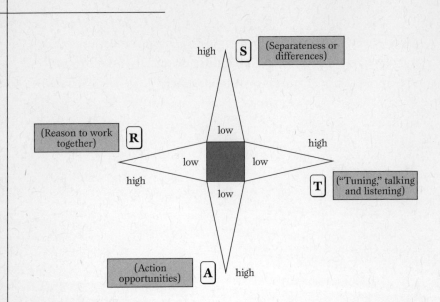

S (separateness) and T (tuning) are necessary to enhance the capacity to generate unforeseen insights and sources of value. S and T operate primarily at the conceptual level. It is through redefining a "fact" or challenging an implicit assumption that new ideas can be created. A (action opportunities) and R (reason to work together) operate primarily at the structural level. It is through action that new players, products, and services actually emerge.

In our work, we found that some of the relationships that were labeled as "generative" by the non-profit social service agency failed to produce anything of value because they were lopsided stars — only a couple of points were well-represented in the relationship.

For example, an ST relationship was one where representatives from the whole community came together to solve a social problem. However, the parties had no reason to work together. They saw themselves as competitors for a shrinking pool of funds, and the trust was not there to see each other as allies. Therefore, there were no real action opportunities defined by the parties.

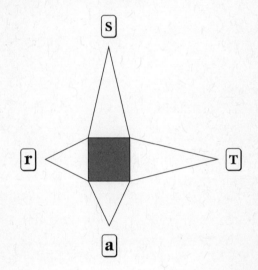

An AR relationship was one where two parties were collaborating to address a problem but the parties were almost "clones." The employees had the same background and perspective. Although they had made time for "T," talking and listening, because they had so few differences, there was little challenge of the status quo.

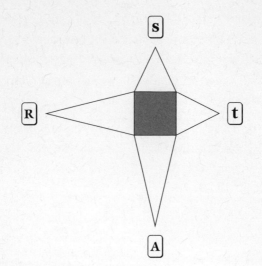

STARs can be fostered within organizations and between organizations. Especially in large organizations, the potential for internal STARs may be high as specialization between departments has increased the capacity for S (separateness or differences). In addition, downsizing may have reduced the time for T (talking and listening to challenge ideas.) Cross-functional task forces address S (separateness or differences) and, if they are well managed, also address T. They also make A (action) a requirement which often makes R (reason to work together) obvious.

Relationships with lots of generative potential have four long points. In complex contexts, these need to be fostered and nurtured. However, there is a down-side. These long STARs require a heavy commitment of time. They can be much more exhausting than relationships with more similarities and less need to explore implicit assumptions. As time is a limited resource, it is important to recognize which relationships need the most generative potential and hence which STARs are more worthwhile. In addition, there is a need to develop and distribute STARs throughout the organization. Trying to centrally control all STARs limits the capacity of the whole organization.

In working with the STAR concept, we often ask groups to identify complex issues for which they need more generative potential in the relationships. Usually we ask them to work through exercises such as the following.

1. Think about your current relationships at work—both inside the organization and outside the organization. What shape of STAR do you see in these relationships? Where do you need to further develop long STARs to address the complex contexts in your work?

2. Mapping current relationship STARs: Identify the key relationships that are engaged in this complex issue. Plot each on the STAR. (The relationships can be with individuals or institutions, and they can be either internal or external to the organization.)

Then we ask, for each relationship, what needs to be done to enhance its generative potential?

To get them started, we often offer a few examples. The lower case letters in the word "STAR" represent the gaps or weaknesses in the relationship.

- A **STaR,** is a relationship with limited action opportunities. What is blocking the action opportunities? Is it a bureaucratic approval process or the need for a supervisor's permission to act?

- A **sTAR** is missing separateness or differences. To enhance its capacity to generate new insights, products, or services, new perspectives need to be brought into the relationship. This may require new participants or at least some structured creativity exercises to reveal hidden assumptions. Who could be added or dropped to enhance the differences in the group?

- A **STar** is all talk and no action. What is preventing the relationship from moving to action? Can you change this context?

- A **stAR** has limited capacity for reflecting on the conceptual changes that are happening. So it may fail to recognize shifts in patterns and thus will expend resources on experiments without capitalizing on the learning from them.

3. Mapping potential relationship STARs—Do the same as the previous exercise but instead of identifying and mapping current relationships, identify potential relationships.

Examples from organizations

(Each of these organizations is a Canadian voluntary sector [not-for-profit] organization. We have disguised the names to provide anonymity.)

National Youth Shelter

National Youth Shelter is one of Canada's largest youth shelters in the country. They provide care and sanctuary and, in addition, focus on advocacy and education for homeless youth. The Toronto chapter wanted to expand their impact by alleviating poverty on a broader scale than their efforts to date. They were aware that the challenge they posed for themselves was complex and needed generative relationships. The STAR was used as a preliminary diagnosis of existing relationships inside and outside the organization. In each case, they found long R but frequently short, or very short, A, T and S attributes.

By examining the S of their board, they were able to articulate the fact that major sectors of society they needed to accomplish their mission were not represented on the board. They also saw how similar the education and vocational backgrounds were of the employees. They made a decision to search out board members, volunteers, and employees with different backgrounds. They realized this would take some time, so in the interim, they sought out the opinions of the missing factions to bring to the staff and board meetings.

They also became aware of how the top-down management style and functionally-based organization limited the T and hence the cross-fertilization of ideas. In addition, they became more aware of how little the Toronto chapter interacted with sister chapters or other homeless advocacy organizations. This was noted as short T and a short A as they felt they were missing opportunities for acting on their mission. Again, specific recommendations were made and followed to engage with others and to collaborate on influencing policy makers and the media to support their cause.

Canadian Cancer Care Foundation
The Canadian Cancer Care Foundation (CCCF) is a registered charitable organization dedicated exclusively to raising funds and to support the advancement of cancer research, education, diagnosis, and treatment. It exists in a highly uncertain environment with increased competition, increased demands for transparency and accountability, changing fund raising practices and donors' attitudes, and policy uncertainty for health charities.

The CCCF used the STAR to examine their relationships with corporations. They felt these relationships needed to have generative potential to help navigate the white waters they were facing in their environment. They decided that these relationships mostly looked like StaRs. Although the differences (S) were great, and the reasons to work together clear (R), they continually let opportunities pass them by (a). The more they discussed this, the more they determined the short "t" was the primary area they needed to work on. They saw the small "a" as somewhat artificial in that there were many opportunities to act, but the lack of tuning in to their differences meant they rarely were able to seize the opportunities in time. They were being "scooped" by the competition on a regular basis.

Others argued that the short "t" was a systemic problem and had led to an organization where staff worked in opposite directions, or at least in isolation, and by so doing had lost the internal cohesion that had once been a hallmark of the organization.

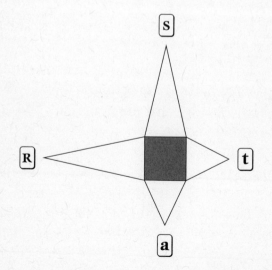

Family Support Agency

The Family Support Agency is an old established organization in Canada that focuses on strengthening families and communities through counseling and community development programs. They used the STAR to evaluate the relationships with their staff, the senior management team, the Board, and with two of their major funders. When they examined the latter, they wanted to learn what they could do to increase the generative potential of their relationships with funders. They invested heavily in both relationships, but they did not feel they were achieving sufficient return or value to their mission given the efforts required. Both of the STARs looked quite similar with long S but all other dimensions were short (or weak). They discussed what it would take to change the "t," "a," and "r" for each relationship. They were quickly discouraged when they examined the first relationship. The power differential was so great and the politics with the funder were so extreme, that they felt it was almost impossible to change the "r" or to work directly on "a." But when they examined the second funding relationship, the energy in the room changed dramatically. They quickly generated a series of options of things they could do to impact "t," "a," and "r."

The question they then posed was where they should focus their opportunity energy. They decided that the first "stuck" relationship would continue to be stuck whether they invested in it or not. However, the second relationship held real potential. They began to list concrete steps, and later acted upon them, to increase the generative potential of their chosen relationship. For the other relationship, they met requirements but did not heavily invest in it with time or energy. In their minds, the relationships were not equal in terms of potential to impact their mission.

Social Service Organization

Social Service Organization (SSO) took pride in their Board. They knew it was diverse, functioned well, and was able to handle serious challenges. One of the Board members brought the STAR concept to their attention. Just out of interest, the Board members decided to each anonymously draw their depiction of the Board's generative potential. The result was a constellation of STARs and all but two looked like the Board needed nothing more to increase its generative potential.

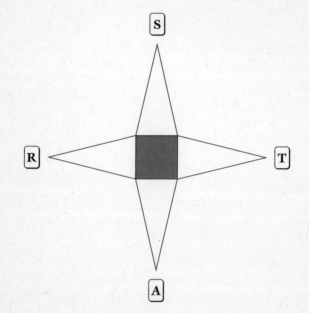

However, two of the STARs were significantly different in the T dimension.

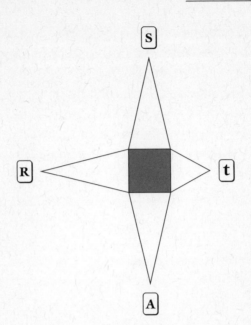

This was a shock to the Board. At first, there was denial. Apparently a couple of the Board members did not understand the tool. But after a while the conversation turned. They began to individually and then collectively identify ways in which they shut down the potential to work with the diversity they had on the Board. The "shut downs" were inadvertent, but real. They decided to bring in a facilitator, versed in diversity, to help them explore ways to tune in better and to reveal the assumptions around the Board table.

Downtown Hospital

Hospitals face a continual challenge of great differences between the clinical specialties and between clinicians and managers. At the Downtown hospital, they determined their staff had an overall profile of StaR—lots of differences, good reasons to work together, but poor tuning and acting on opportunities. They saw the long S as both a threat and an opportunity for the hospital to have a significant impact on the health of the community.

Downtown Hospital talked about being patient centered. This was a value shared by both clinical staff and management staff. When some of the management staff were exposed to the STAR concept, they decided that with busy, and often impatient, clinicians, working on the poor "t" directly would not be feasible. Instead, they determined that they would be won over by actions. They began to identify actions where emergent, generative potential was demonstrated and they then talked about how the successes were generated. They looked for initiatives they could support across the disciplines and the other hospital divides. These were often small action opportunities but they created energy—a buzz. When the buzz spread, they then had the attention of individual or small groups of clinicians and staff members. They were then able to work on the "t" dimension more directly. They could emphasize the strength of the differences when they were used to find new ways of acting. They used actions to create momentum and then back into the tuning dimension.

Conclusions

The concept of generative relationships is appealing. The idea of creating something that is more than the sum of the parts is indeed a draw for most people struggling with complex human system issues. However, the concept is too vague or too conceptual for most people to use to good effect in achieving their missions. We have found that the STAR diagram is a useful way to focus people's attention on the different dimensions that contribute to a generative relationship. The STAR is not perfect. It does, however, allow for new questions and insights to emerge. The examples above used the STAR to:

1. Differentiate the amount of energy to invest into relationships.

2. Examine whether relationships are judged the same by all involved.

3. Discern where efforts need to be made to have greatest impact on the relationship's generative potential.

We believe the greatest value of the STAR is its capacity to reframe the focus of conversations about relationships.

Brenda J. Zimmerman, Ph.D., M.B.A.

Dr. Brenda Zimmerman is a professor of Strategic Management at the Schulich School of Business at York University in Toronto. During 2000–2002, she joined McGill's Faculty of Management as an Associate Professor and had a joint appointment with the Faculty of Medicine. Between 1998–2003, she was a professor in the McGill-McConnell Masters' Program for Voluntary Sector Leaders.

Her primary research applies complexity science to management and leadership issues in organizations, especially voluntary sector or not-for-profit organizations, experiencing high levels of uncertainty and turbulence. Since 1996 the bulk of her research and teaching has focused on health care with an emphasis on clinicians in management and leadership roles. She has been an invited speaker at many health care conferences in the USA sponsored by the American Hospital Association, VHA (Voluntary Hospital Association), and the Veterans Hospital Association as well as a number of not-for-profit health care systems. She has written many articles, book chapters, and a book on the topic of complexity and management in health care.

She received her B.S. from the University of Toronto in Ontario, Canada, and her M.B.A. and Ph.D. from York University.

Bryan Hayday, M.A.

Bryan Hayday's career spans roles as a CEO, Executive Director, lecturer, and consultant with government and non-governmental agencies and organizations in the health, education, and social service sectors across Canada. Frequent assignments in scenario planning, organizational change, strategic management, leadership development, and governance issues characterize Bryan's consulting practice. Through this work, he increasingly uses the frameworks of complex adaptive systems as the basis for practical recommendations that derive from robust strategies. In addition to his consulting practice, Bryan is part of the Non-Profit Management and Leadership Program at the Schulich School of Business at York University, teaching courses on organizational development, leadership, and complexity.

A graduate of both York University and Loyola College (Montreal) in Inter-Disciplinary Studies, Bryan's early career included work in organizational development and mental health consultation.

Brian is currently Principal Consultant for ChangeAbility, Inc.

For more information on the work and research conducted through ChangeAbility Inc., you are invited to visit the website at www.change-ability.ca.

Bibliography

Accelerated Schools Project. (2003). (Retrieved from http://www.acceleratedschools.net, February 26, 2003).

Ahmad Z. Hammad. (1996). *The Opening to The Quran.* Illinois: Quranic Literacy Institute.

Al-Faruqi, Isma'il Raji. *Meta-Religion: A Framework For Islamic Moral Theology.* Washington: Islamic Institute for Strategic Studies. Policy Paper No. 5, June, 2000.

Allington, R. (2002). *Big Brother and the National Reading Curriculum: How Ideology Trumped Evidence.* Portsmouth, NH: Heinemann.

Al-Qoz, Anas Abdul-Hameed. (2000). *Men and the Universe: Reflections of Idn Al-Qayyem.* Riyadh: Darussalam.

Anon. (1998). Carriacou and Petite Martinique Integrated Physical Development and Environmental Management Plan (Planning for Sustainable Development). Government of Grenada, UNDP, UNCHS and CDB.

Berkes, F., R. Mahon, P. McConney, R. Pollnac & R. Pomeroy. (2001). *Managing Small-Scale Fisheries: Alternative Directions and Methods.* Ottawa, Canada: IDRC.

Bolman, L. & T. Deal.(1997). *Reframing Organizations: Artistry, Choice and Leadership.* San Francisco: Jossey-Bass/Pfeiffer.

Briggs, J. & F.D. Peat. (1989). *Turbulent Mirror: An Illustrated Guide to Chaos Theory and the Science Of Wholeness.* NY: Harper and Row.

Canada/SVG Fisheries Development Project. (1992). "Community and fishing profiles of Canouan, Paget Farm, Ashton, Clifton, and Kingstown Beach: Report of Baseline Data Studies." Volume III: *St. Vincent and the Grenadines Community Profiles:* Fisheries Division.

Carlson, D. & M. Apple. (1998). *Power, Knowledge, Pedagogy: the Meaning of Democratic Education in Unsettling Times.* Boulder, Colorado: Westview Press.

Carroll, L. (1866). *Alice's Adventures in Wonderland.* London: Macmillan & Co.

Chakalall, Y. S., R. Mahon & H. A. Oxenford. (In press). *Activities of Trading Vessels and Supplying Fishers in the Grenadine Islands, Lesser Antilles.* Proceedings of the Gulf & Caribbean Fisheries Institute.

Cohen, J. & I. Stewart. (1994). *The Collapse of Chaos: Discovering Simplicity in a Complex World.* NY: Penguin Books.

Cowan, G., D. Pines & D. Meltzer. (1994). *Complexity: Metaphors, Models, and Reality.* Reading, Massachusetts: Addison-Wesley Publishing Company.

Darling-Hammond, L. (1997). *The Right to Learn: A Blueprint for Creating Schools that Work.* San Francisco : Jossey-Bass.

Dewey, J.(1997). *How We Think.* Dover Publications.

Dooley, K. (1996). "A Complex Adaptive Systems Model of Organizational Change." *Nonlinear Dynamics, Psychology, and Life Sciences,* 1(1), 69–97.

Eoyang, G., E. Olson & G. Kennedy. *Complexity 101: Concepts and Tools for OD Practitioners.* Unpublished manuscript. p. 6.

Eoyang, G. (1997). *Coping with Chaos: Seven Simple Tools.* Cheyenne, Wyoming: Legumo Publishing.

Eoyang, G. *Conditions for Self-organizing in Human Systems.* Unpublished Ph.D. Dissertation, The Union Institute and University; December 28, 2001; viii,x,xi, 11.

Freire, P. & D. Macedo. (1998). *Teachers As Cultural Workers: Letters to Those Who Dare Teach (Edge. Critical Studies in Educational Theory.)* Boulder, Colorado: Westview Press.

Gharajedaghi, J. (1990). *Systems Thinking: Managing Chaos and Complexity.* Butterworth-Heinemann.

Gladwell, M. (2000). The Tipping Point. Boston: Little, Brown and Co.

Goldstein, J. (1994). *The Unshackled Organization.* New York: Productivity Press.

Hollingsworth, S. (1994). *Teacher Research and Urban Literacy Education : Lessons and Conversations in a Feminist Key.* New York : Teachers College Press.

Hopfenberg, W. A., H. M. Levin and Associates. (1993). *The Accelerated Schools Resource Guide.* San Francisco: Jossey-Bass.

Jenkins, J. & M. Jenkins. (1997). *The Social Process Triangles.* Imaginal Training.

Karen Harding. (1994). "Causality Then and Now: Al Ghazali and Quantum Theory." *American Journal of Islamic Social Sciences,* 10:2.

Lakoff, G. & M. Johnson. (1980). *Metaphors We Live By.* Chicago: University of Chicago Press.

Lane, David & Robert Maxfield. (1996). "Strategy Under Complexity: Fostering Generative Relationships," *Long Range Planning,* Vol. 29, No. 2, pp. 215-231.

Lewis, R. & B. Regine. (2000). *The Soul at Work: Complexity Theory and Business.* New York: Simon & Schuster.

Lissack, M. & J. Roos. (1999). *The Next Common Sense: Mastering Corporate Complexity through Coherence.* London: Nicholas Brealey Publishing Limited.

Luft, J. (1984). *Group Processes: An Introduction to Group Dynamics.* Mayfield Publishing.

McDaniel, R. (2002). "Making the Leap to Organizations." P. Buscell (Ed.). *Emerging.* Plexus Institute. Sept.–Oct. p. 11.

Mermer, Yamine B. (1996). *Induction, Science and Causation: Some Critical Reflections.* Islamabad: Islamic Research Institute.

Morowitz, H. (2003). *The Emergence of Everything.* NY: Oxford University Press.

Murata, Sachiko & William Chittick. (1996). *The Moral Vision of Islam.* London: I.B. Tauris & Co. Ltd.

Nasr, Seyyed H. (1981). *Islamic Life and Thought.* Albany: State University of New York Press.

OECS. 1991. *'Principles of Environmental Sustainability in the OECS' St. Georges Declaration of 2001.* Organization of Eastern Caribbean States, St. Lucia: The Morne.

Olson, E. & G. Eoyang (2001). *Facilitating Organization Change: Lessons from Complexity Science.* San Francisco: Jossey-Bass/Pfeiffer.

Olson, E. & G. Eoyang. (2001). "Using Complexity Science to Facilitate Self-organizing Processes in Teams." *OD Practitioner.* 33.3. p. 38.

Oshry, B. (1996). *Seeing Systems: Unlocking the Mysteries of Organizational Life.* San Francisco: Berrett-Kohler.

Patterson, L. & F. Mallow. (2001). *Teaching Every Child, a Guide for Literacy Teams, Grades 1–3.* Christopher-Gordon Publishers, Inc.

Senge, P. (1990). *The Fifth Discipline; The Art and Practice of the Learning Organization.* New York: Doubleday Currency.

Silverstein, S. (1974). *Where the Sidewalk Ends.* New York: Harper & Row. p. 112.

Stacey, R. (2001). *Complex Responsive Processes in Organizations: Learning and Knowledge Creation.* London: Routledge.

Stacey, R., D. Griffin & P. Shaw. (2000). *Complexity and Management: Fad Or Radical Challenge to Systems Thinking?* London: Routledge.

Stacey, R. (1992). *Managing the Unknowable: Strategic Boundaries Between Order and Chaos In Organizations.* San Francisco: Jossey-Bass.

Stewart, I. & J. Cohen. (1999). *Figments of Reality.* New York: Cambridge University Press.

Taylor, B., P.D. Pearson, K. Clark & S. Walpole. (1999) *Beating the Odds in Teaching All Children to Read.* CIERA Report #2-006. University of Michigan, Ann Arbor: Center for the Improvement of Early Reading Achievement.

Texas Education Agency (Retrieved from http://www.tea.state.tx.us/ on February 26, 2003.)

Tovani, C. & E. O. Keene. (2000). *I Read It but I Don't Get It: Comprehension Strategies for Adolescent Readers.* Portland, ME: Stenhouse Publishers.

Waldrop, M.M. (1992). *Complexity: The Emerging Science at the Edge of Order and Chaos.* London: Penguin.

Weick, K. (1979). *The Social Psychology of Organizing.* Reading, Massachusetts: Addison-Wesley.

Wheatley, M. J. (1994). *Leadership and the New Science: Learning About Organization from an Orderly Universe.* San Francisco: Barrett-Koehler.

Wickstrom, C. & J. Curtis. (2002). "Creating Space for an Informed Literacy Teacher When the School District Adopts a Scripted Phonics Program." Annual Conference of the College Reading Association.

Zimmerman, Brenda & Curt Lindberg, Paul Plsek. (1998). *Edgeware: Insights from Complexity Science for Health Care Leaders.* Irving, Texas: VHA Inc.

Zimmerman, Brenda J. & Bryan C. Hayday. (1999). "A Board's Journey Into Complexity Science," *Group Decision Making and Negotiation.* Vol. 8.

Introducing the Human Systems Dynamics Institute

Where do turbulence, change, and upheaval come from?

What can I do about them?

When will they stop so I my world gets back to normal?

Even people who like change feel overwhelmed by the current speed and turbulence that challenge individuals, teams, and organizations. Old stories, tools, and techniques that helped in the past don't work any more. Change comes too fast from too many directions all at the same time.

A new science is emerging at the intersection between complexity and social sciences. Human systems dynamics (HSD) integrates the age-old wisdom about social systems with cutting-edge discoveries in the new, nonlinear physical sciences. The result is a powerful new way to think and act productively in human systems.

The Human Systems Dynamics Institute facilitates the development of theory and practice in human systems dynamics. It includes:

- A membership network of practitioners and researchers who are developing innovative theory and practice in the field.

- A press that publishes books and training materials to support dissemination of emerging questions and discoveries.

- A service bureau to link members with clients who want to use HSD principles and techniques to improve individual and organizational performance.

- A foundation that invests in research and experimental practice in the field.

For more information about the HSD Institute or to get involved in its programs and services, visit the website at www.hsdinstitute.org.

Voices from the Field is the first publication of the HSD Institute Press. We expect future titles to reflect the best thinking and action of those exploring the landscape of complex human systems. You are invited to join the conversation, contact the authors, and contribute your own insights. To participate in this on-going, self-organizing process, visit the website and get connected!

Index